D0421085

Milady's
Black
Cosmetology

Thomas Hayden and James Williams

Mi
(A Division of Delmar Publishers, Inc.)
3 Columbia Circle, Box 15015
Albany, NY 12212-5015

Art Director:	John P. Fornieri
Production Manager:	Jan M. Lavin
Graphic Artists:	Pat Miret
	Mark Stein
	Pat Genova
	Roberto Williams
Typesetters:	Barbara Cardillo
	Paul Gafton
Illustrators:	Shiz Horii, Ed Tadiello
Cover Photograph:	Steven Landis
Text Photographs:	Michael Gallitelli
	Eric Von Lockhart
	Steven Landis
Photo credits on page 54:	Hair by Garland Drake International: Keiko Shino
	Makeup by Dianne O
	Photo by Robert Lynden, Los Angeles, CA

10   9   8   7   6

Acknowledgments

Milady Publishing Company extends grateful acknowledgment to the following individuals who contributed to the development of this book:

Phyllis Causey - Black Hair, Inc., Los Angles, California

Elizabeth Daniel - Hempstead, New York

Linda Fine - Fine Concepts, Inc., Easton, Connecticut

Pegi Males-Hills - Bloomingdale, Ohio

Carolyn Perrin - Robert Fiance Hair Design Institute, New York New York

Mary Jane Tenerelli - New York, New York

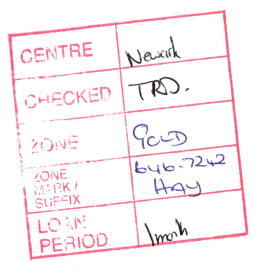

Contents

Sharp Lines
 and
Soft Curls
Shape
The 90's Look

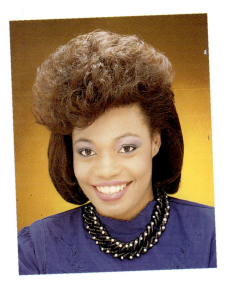

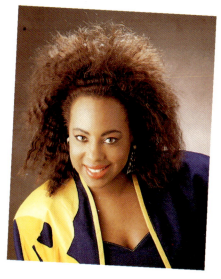

Savvy
Silhouettes
Suitable
Styles

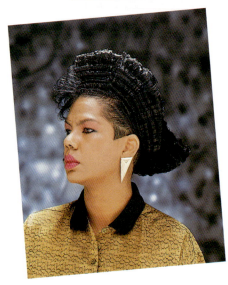

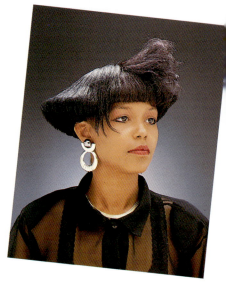

A Splash
of
Color

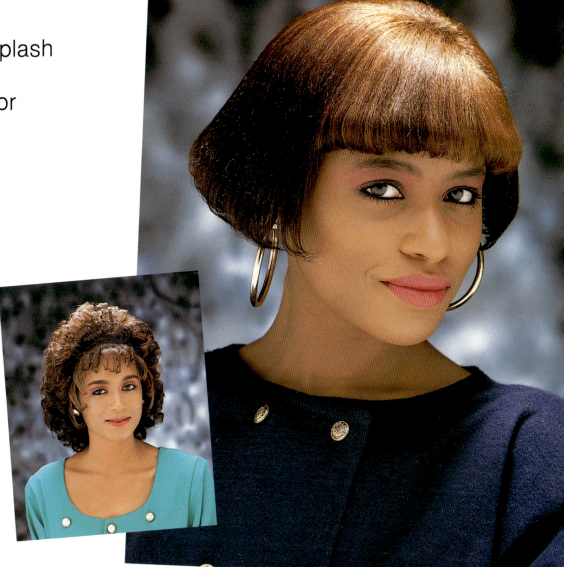

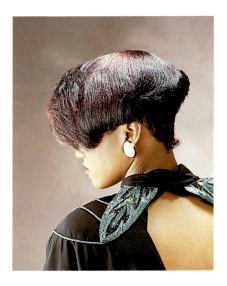

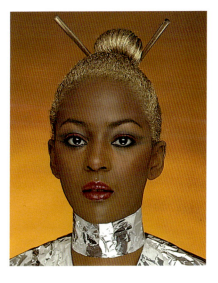

The New
Fashion
Accessory
Hair
Extensions!

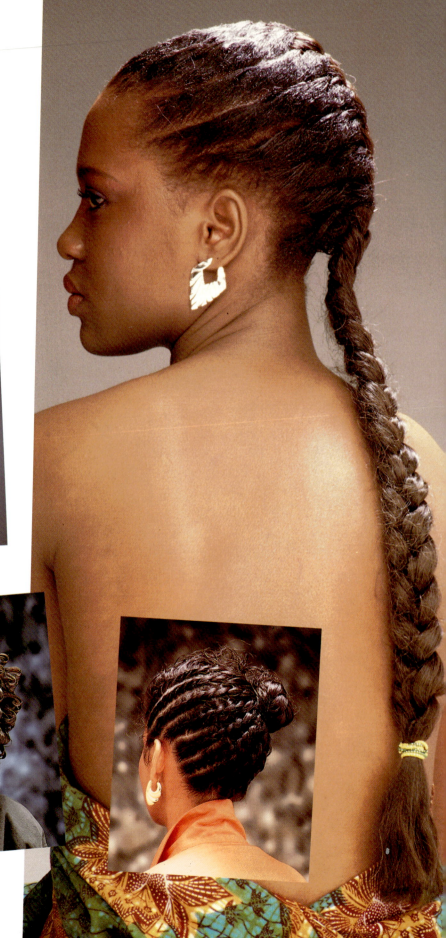

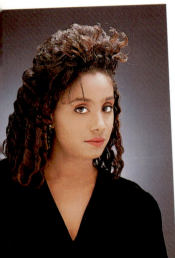

Introduction

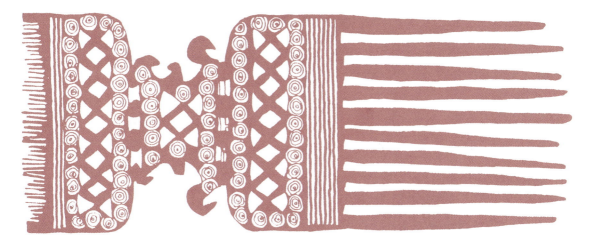

A HISTORY OF BLACK STYLING

The practice of Black cosmetology dates to ancient times. Thousands of years ago in Africa, intricate combs were carved and used to groom Black hair. Hair was styled and ornamented with clay, beads, flowers, ribbons and combs. Braiding was often symbolic and could, for example, indicate if a woman was single, in mourning, or a high priestess. In some tribes the length of a woman's hair was a measure of her strength.

In some superstitious tribes, it was believed that good and bad spirits entered the body through the hair and that cutting the hair was the only way to drive them away. Other tribes had the hair hang over the shoulders during religious rituals to allow evil spirits to escape. After a ceremonial dance, the long hair was cut in the tribe's distinctive fashion.

Many tribes are still identified by their hairstyles. The Masai women of Kenya wind long hair into an elaborate clubbed bob). The men of Kenya wear ornamental combs and tie brightly colored bands around their heads (Figure I-1). The Zulus have always maintained a distinctive hairstyle original to their tribe: clay-coated ringlets twisted and brought down low over the forehead and neck.

Half Heads was the name given to the royal runners of the Dahomey Empire. They shaved one side of the head and carefully shaped the other in a style closely resembling the American version of the Afro.

From the 1700s through the Civil War, Black slaves in America were permitted little or no access to the means to groom and style hair. Without combs, shampoo, nets, pins, scissors, and the like, Black slaves had little choice but to cover their heads in rags or hack off their hair as best they could, as close to the head as possible, with crude implements like farm shears. Scalp disease and hair damage were prevalent. With the abolishment of slavery came the reinstatement of healthy, fashionable hair for Blacks. Many Blacks became cosmetologists and salon owners catering exclusively to a Black clientele.

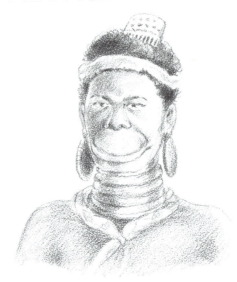

Figure I-1. Masai hairstyle

The credit for real progress in the field of Black cosmetology in the late 1800s and through the 1920s goes to two pioneering women, Annie M. Turnbo Malone and Madame C. J. Walker. Ms. Malone created one of the first scalp and hair treatments for Black hair and called it *Wonderful Hair Grower*. Its purpose was to smooth overly curly hair. Her business grew until she had amassed several million dollars and had created a chain of beauty schools that specifically taught Black cosmetology. She had a troop of agents who went door to door and sold her cosmetic preparations across the country. Ms. Malone was one of the first to turn Black beauty culture into an industry in America.

Madame C. J. Walker also developed a hair products empire that became very successful and made her one of the first Black millionaires. She developed a hot comb to straighten curly hair that replaced the dangerous and damaging method of applying lard to the scalp and then pulling or ironing hair wrapped in heated rags. Mme. Walker's hot comb was used in conjunction with an oily hair pomade she created, which protected the hair as well as weighting it down to further remove curl. Mme. Walker eventually owned a manufacturing plant, beauty salons, and a chain of schools that taught the Walker method of cosmetology. She, like Ms. Malone, had a sales force of women who sold her products and taught her methods door to door.

The Walker methods of straightening and styling black hair were reflected in the fingerwaves and short bobs of the 1920s (Figure I-2). Later variations were the *Betty Boop* and "poodle curl" looks of the 1930s. To keep hair sleek, women as well as men wore stocking caps to bed.

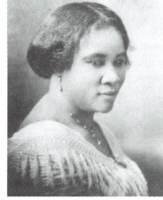

Figure I-2.
Madam C.J. Walker, began a Black hair care empire in 1905.

2

The bob and fingerwaves were popular in the roaring twenties.

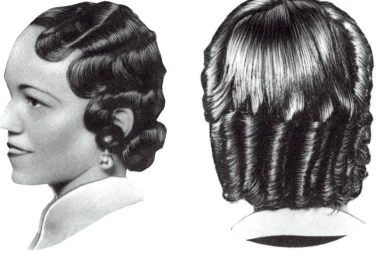

In the 1940s barbershops and beauty salons for Black clients were everywhere. They offered press and curls, straightening and marcel waves. Popular hairstyles for women were exemplified by stars such as jazz and blues singer Billie Holiday (Figure I-3).

Figure I-3. Jazz singer Billie Holiday in a popular 1940s hairsyle.

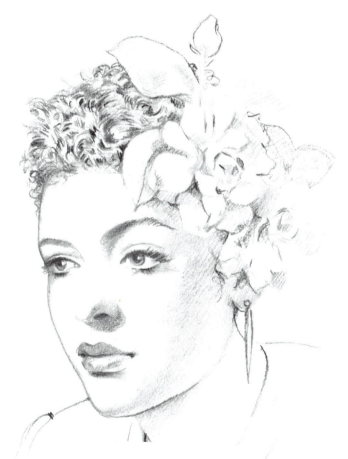

Favorite styles were smooth, relaxed looks with hair rolled away from the face and the back of the head. Braids and upsweep styles were also popular.

At the end of the 1950s, popular press and curl hairstyles were the ponytail, structured flip, and page boy as well as the French roll. Wigs were popular and the Motown influence was strong. Modified bush and high pompadour looks were in demand in barbershops.

In the early 1960s many Black men opted for a very short, close look in hair. A man would put a little pomade on his hair and slip a stocking cap on overnight to force curls into waves. If he didn't like the short cut, *conked* or relaxed hair was a fashionable alternative. The in look for women in the early sixties was teased and bouffant coiffures. Shorter styles had front and side curls or waves with waxed napes. By the late sixties Blacks were letting their hair grow out naturally in versions of the Afro (Figure I-4). Men turned away from stocking caps and processing equipment and let their hair curl.

Figure I-4. The Afro hairstyle popular in the late 1960s as men turned toward a natural look.

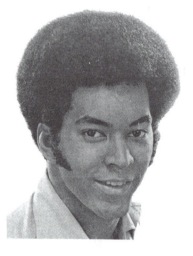

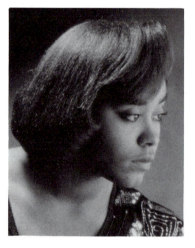

Chemically relaxed hairstyles.

By the early seventies chemically relaxed hairstyles were once again popular. New brands of relaxers gave styling freedom to shag cuts, flips, and bangs. Soft curl permanents were suddenly in wide demand. The Afro became more versatile with puffs, geometric cuts, and even some splashes of color. Then the Afro was joined with braids and cornrows.

The ancient art of cornrowing (canerow to West Indians) became very popular again at this time. It offered unlimited and dramatic alternatives in Black styling. It also helped people with thinning hair. The cosmetologist would cornrow the remaining natural hair of the client and then weave in new, usually synthetic, hair (Figure I-5).

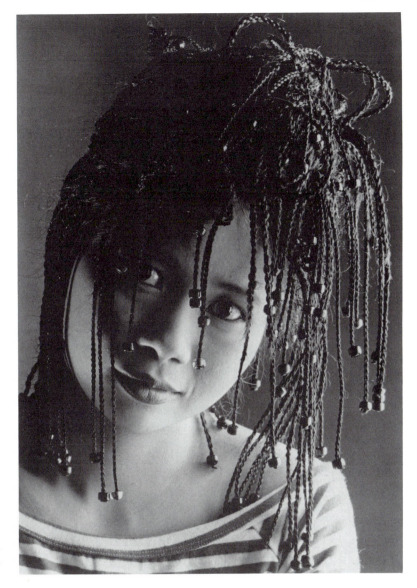

Figure I-5. A synthetic cornrow style. Photo courtesy of Maureen Fielding.

Black hairstyling for the eighties included three-dimensional coloring and asymmetrical curls. The basic bob continues to be popular worldwide. It can be worn crimped, waved or completely straight with the help of chemical relaxers. Today's cosmetologist has a wealth of products at his or her fingertips. Creativity is enhanced by the availability of soft curl perms, relaxers, hair coloring products, and styling agents such as mousse and gel. Improved chemicals as well as a diverse wealth of heritages to draw upon have made choices in Black hair design both unique and beautiful.

Chapter 1 Brushing and Combing

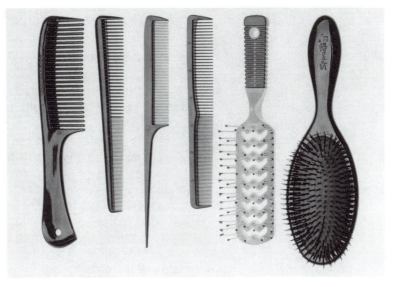

LEARNING OBJECTIVES

After you have mastered this chapter, you will be able to:

1. Explain what must be determined before brushing or combing Black hair.
2. List five reasons to avoid brushing the Black client's hair.
3. Give the procedure for brushing Black hair.
4. Give the procedure for combing Black hair.

INTRODUCTION

Because of its density, texture and curl configuration, the Black client's hair can break more easily than Caucasian hair. Caution then must be exercised when brushing or combing Black hair.

SPECIAL CONSIDERATIONS IN BRUSHING AND COMBING

Many Black clients rely on chemical services such as relaxing and soft curl perming to keep their hair manageable. The regrowth at the scalp will be a different texture from the rest of the hair. Each section must be separately considered when brushing and combing.

You will have to determine the following:

- If the client's hair has been chemically relaxed, soft curl permed, pressed, or left in its natural state.
- If the hair warrants brushing, combing, or both.
- What service you are about to perform.

BRUSHING

Brushing distributes the oils from the scalp throughout the hair. Brushing also stimulates oil and lymph glands and increases circulation.

When to Brush

Brushing is advisable:

1. If the client's hair and scalp are excessively dry. Brushing will stimulate oil production and distribute the oils throughout the hair.
2. To evenly distribute products such as pomade.
3. As a styling technique to remove roller lines after a set.

When Not to Brush Do **not** brush the client's hair:

1. When there is more than one curl configuration on the same head (example: excessive regrowth).
2. Before a chemical service. Brushing might cause the scalp to be overly sensitive to the chemicals.
3. Directly after a chemical service. At this time hair must be treated very gently.
4. If the client does not regularly brush his or her hair at home. Unbrushed hair will be too fragile for vigorous brushing. You might break the hair.
5. When the client's hair is wet. When hair is stretched to its maximum length, it is much too fragile to be brushed.

Types of Brushes Brush selection is very important, especially if the hair is fragile or dense. Whenever possible, use a natural bristle brush. This type of brush is the least likely to damage the Black client's hair. Vent brushes are excellent for detangling (Figure 1-1). Bristles should be slanted and/or rounded. They must never be cut straight across. This could tear the client's hair.

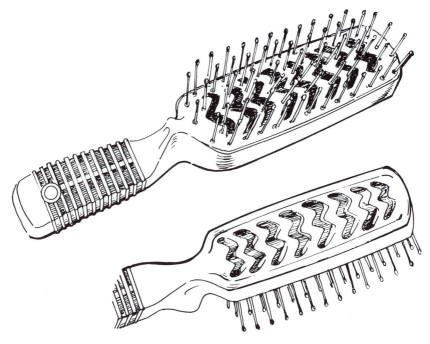

Figure 1-1. Vent brush

Never use a brush designed for wigs on the client's hair. Always avoid using a round brush to brush through the client's hair. These are used only as styling tools.

Because of the density of the client's hair, the bristles must be long, firm, and widely spaced if they are to penetrate the hair's thickness.

Procedure for Brushing

1. Remove hair ornaments.
2. Detangle with a wide-tooth comb.
3. Section the hair into four parts: forehead to nape; ear to ear.
4. Work forward starting at the nape. Hair at the nape usually has the tightest curl pattern, which makes it the most difficult to brush. It is not necessary to brush briskly. Always use a gentle, but firm, touch.
5. Brush gently, in sections, until you reach the forehead.
6. Take the brush and begin brushing in 1/2-inch sections using your other hand to hold the hair you are not brushing out of your way.
7. Brush downward. Never use reverse brushing -- it will tangle the client's hair and can cause breakage.
8. Hold the ends of long hair taut to stretch out the curls and protect hair while brushing.

COMBING

You'll have to master combing if you are to detangle sections, make partings, and style the Black client's hair.

Detangling

Detangling is the first step in every professional service you will perform on the Black client. Excessively curly hair must be detangled carefully and gently due to its fragile composition.

You will need the following combs:

1. **Detangling comb.** This is a wide-tooth comb with smooth, heavy teeth molded into an *S*-pattern. Teeth should be spaced approximately 1/8 inch apart. This comb usually has two rows of teeth (Figure 1-2).
2. **Basic wide-tooth comb.** This may be used as long as there is sufficient space between the teeth. This comb usually has only one row of teeth (Figure 1-3).

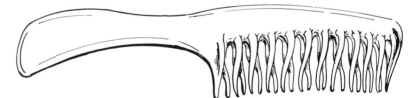

Figure 1-2. Detangler comb

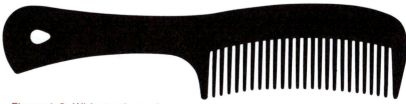

Figure 1-3. Wide-tooth comb

9

3. **Pick.** This is a flexible plastic tool with long, thin teeth that are widely spaced (Figure 1-4).

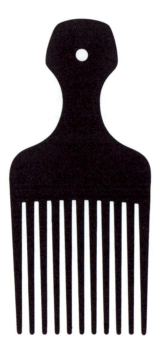

Figure 1-4. Pick

> *Caution:* Never use a conventional comb with teeth that are close together. This will damage the Black client's hair.

Procedure for Detangling You will be working with either wet or dry hair depending on what service you are going to perform.

> *Caution:* The pick is only to be used as a detangler on wet hair. Since the Black client's hair is more elastic when wet, the flexibility of the pick might stretch the dry hair to its breaking point.

1. Section the hair into four parts: ear to ear; forehead to nape.
2. Starting at the nape, make 1/2-inch partings. Comb gently from scalp to ends.
3. Work forward from the nape, section by section, holding the hair taut and combing downward.

> *Note:* Always work up from ends, 1/4 inch at a time.

Sectioning   To section the Black client's hair for styling, perming, and so on, you will need a fantail comb. This comb should be made of hard rubber. Use only the tail portion to divide the hair into sections. The close spacing of the teeth often makes this comb unsuitable for Black hair. The client's choice of style and service will determine your comb selection.

Relaxed hair: Wide-tooth comb, standard straight comb, fantail comb (Figure 1-5)

Soft curl perm: Pick for lifting and separating, detangling comb, wide-tooth comb for forming waves, standard straight comb (Figure 1-6)

Natural hair: Pick for lifting and separating, detangling comb, wide-tooth comb

Figure 1-5. Fantail comb

Figure 1-6. Standard straight comb

QUESTIONS FOR   1. What things must be determined before brushing and combing
REVIEW   Black hair?

2. What are five reasons to avoid brushing the Black client's hair?

3. What is the procedure for brushing Black hair?

4. What is the procedure for combing Black hair?

Chapter 2 Shampooing

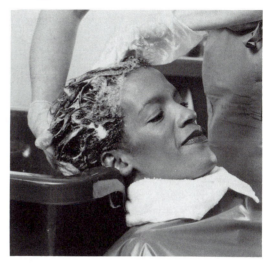

LEARNING OBJECTIVES

After you have mastered this chapter, you will be able to:

1. Name four shampooing considerations.
2. Describe the shampoo that should be used on chemically relaxed hair.
3. Give the correct procedure for shampooing Black hair.

INTRODUCTION

The Black client's hair is often fragile due to chemical services so it is very important that the right type of shampoo and the correct shampooing technique are used. The following chapter will outline the shampoos and the procedure you should apply for this hair type.

SHAMPOOING CONSIDERATIONS

The items below need to be taken into consideration before the shampoo to be used on a Black client is chosen.

1. **How often does the client shampoo his or her hair?** Often, clients with excessively curly hair shampoo less. This hair is sometimes drier and more fragile and cannot withstand daily washing. Many Black clients return to the salon each week for a shampoo and styling.

2. **What sort of relaxing service (if any) was performed on the client's hair?** Check to see if the hair has been relaxed. Ask the client how it was done. Was a hot comb or press used, or was the hair chemically relaxed?

3. **What is the client's daily hair care procedure?** Does he or she use oils or conditioners daily? Does he or she use a hot comb every day to touch up areas where the hair has reverted back to its natural curl pattern? If the hair has been chemically relaxed, determine the amount of time between touch-ups, and if the hair has been conditioned, the amount of time between treatments.

4. **Is the client's hair curly?** You'll have to determine if the hair is naturally curly or if the curl has been re-formed with a soft curl permanent wave.

> **Note:** Once you have determined what has been done to the client's hair, find out what service the client is requesting at this time. The selection of the shampoo product might be determined by the service you are about to perform.

Preparation for Shampoo

1. Select and arrange materials. You will need the following:
   - towels
   - wide-tooth comb
   - shampoo
   - conditioner
2. Seat the client and drape.
3. Remove hair ornaments and earrings.
4. Examine the condition of the hair and scalp.
5. Comb through the hair with a wide-tooth comb.
6. Take a subsection of the hair and hold it taut with one hand (Figure 2-1).

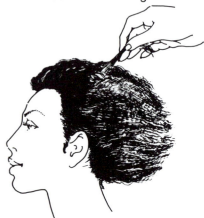

Figure 2-1. Hold subsection taut.

7. Gently comb through with the other hand (working from scalp to ends). This technique prevents breakage and eliminates client discomfort.
8. Adjust the chair so that the client is comfortable.

SHAMPOO SELECTION

Your shampoo selection will depend upon the services already performed on the client, as well as the one that you are about to perform.

Physically Relaxed Hair

For hair physically relaxed by pressing or silking, use a shampoo for normal hair. Hair that has been pressed or silked has been treated with oils and pomades. The shampoo must be strong enough to break down and cleanse away the residue from these oils, yet not damage the hair. Shampoos for oily hair are too harsh for physically relaxed hair.

Soft Curled Hair

For hair with a soft curl permanent wave, use a gentle, nondrying formula. Check the manufacturer's instructions since many soft curl permanent kits come with their own shampoo, or indicate what shampoo to use. Your instructor may advise that you use the same product line.

Natural Hair

For hair that has not been processed, use a shampoo according to the condition and texture. Natural hair is usually also dry. Your instructor can help you analyze this hair type.

THE SHAMPOO SERVICE   The same shampoo procedure is used on all types of Black hair. Always keep the condition of the hair in mind.

Procedure for Shampooing

1. Adjust the water so that it is warm and comfortable for your client.
2. Wet the hair thoroughly. Most Black client's hair is very dense, and depending on previous services, it might be extremely porous. Water is readily absorbed. It will take several minutes to thoroughly saturate the client's hair. Continue to wet the hair until it is completely saturated.
3. Generously apply the shampoo that is indicated by the condition of the hair. Add shampoo until you have a slight lather. Due to the density and porosity of the Black client's hair, you might have to add more shampoo.
4. Section the hair with your fingers, and massage the shampoo lather at the scalp. This is very important. This is where you will find a buildup of oil and residue from styling aids. You'll have to break down this oil, and cleanse the scalp area. Massage briskly to release the residue. Work from the front hairline to the nape and then from side to side (Figures 2-2 and 2-3).

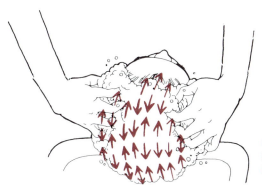

Figure 2-2. Manipulate the scalp from hairline at ears to the top of the head.

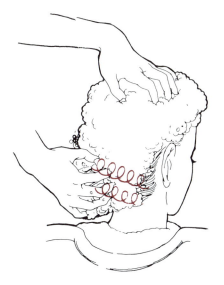

Figure 2-3. Lift the client's head to shampoo the nape area.

15

5. When every area of the scalp has been thoroughly cleansed, work the shampoo through the hair to the ends.

> *Caution:* Exert massage pressure only at the scalp area. Be gentle when working shampoo through the hair to the ends, especially if the client's hair is fragile and easily damaged.

6. Rinse hair thoroughly. Keep rinsing until the water is clear and free from shampoo. Make sure all the shampoo has been removed from the scalp area.
7. Repeat steps 4 through 6.
8. Towel blot and gently wrap the client's hair; then return the client to the styling area.
9. Using a clean, wide-tooth comb, gently detangle the client's hair. Begin at the ends and, holding the hair taut in one hand, work up the subsection to the scalp. Never pull or tug.

QUESTIONS FOR REVIEW

1. What four questions should be considered before a shampoo is given?
2. What are the characteristics of shampoo used on chemically relaxed hair?
3. What is the correct procedure for shampooing Black hair?

Chapter 3 Conditioning

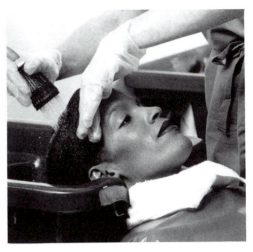

LEARNING OBJECTIVES

After you have mastered this chapter, you will be able to:
1. Give the benefits of instant and penetrating conditioners.
2. Give the procedure for a penetrating conditioner.
3. Name the three types of moisturizers and explain how each works.
4. Explain how to condition dry, damaged hair that has undergone a chemical service.
5. Give the 12 movements for scalp massage.
6. Explain the best way to get to know the product line of conditioners you will be recommending to clients.

INTRODUCTION

Conditioning, moisturizing, and scalp treatments are very important for Black clients who have excessively dry hair or scalps or for those who have undergone chemical services such as soft curl perming or chemical relaxing. Many Black clients will have hair with a thick cuticle layer, which impedes the flow of the natural oils that keep hair soft and supple. Thick, curly hair can also be difficult to thoroughly brush, and clients with this type of hair will miss out on the beneficial scalp stimulation that regular brushing provides. Yet hair textures and curl patterns will vary widely among Black clients and so you must carefully examine the hair and scalp of each individual before recommending conditioning and scalp treatments.

CONDITIONERS

Conditioners come in two forms: penetrating and instant. Penetrating types can be used before or after chemical services as well as on virgin hair. Instant types are used after a shampoo or chemical service. Penetrating conditioners are absorbed into the cortex of the hair and repair damage such as excess porosity and overall weakness of the hair shaft. Instant conditioners coat the hair shaft, flattening ruffled cuticles and giving the hair a healthier, shinier, bouncier appearance and making it easier to comb and style. Conditioners are the cosmetologist's main weapon against dry, lifeless hair and split ends.

Penetrating Conditioners

Penetrating conditioners are composed of animal proteins. These proteins are refined so that their molecules are small enough to penetrate the hair shaft, moving into the cortex and strengthening the hair and making it softer and more supple in appearance. This type of conditioner can be used before or after a chemical treatment. Using a penetrating conditioner once a week will keep your client's hair in optimum condition. Always follow the manufacturer's directions when using a penetrating conditioner. Some products may call for the use of a plastic cap or a cool dryer to facilitate penetration. Be guided by your instructor.

Procedure for Penetrating Conditioning

1. Determine the overall condition of the scalp and hair.
2. Shampoo the hair.
3. Part the hair into four sections, from nose to nape and from ear to ear.
4. Apply conditioner section by section with a tint brush. Massage conditioner gently into hair (Figure 3-1).

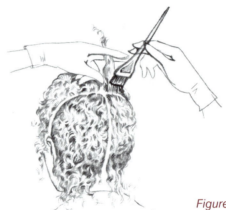

Figure 3-1. Apply conditioner.

5. Concentrate on the dry areas, especially the ends and nape where hair is most resistant to processing.
6. If the product in use requires the client to wear a cap, place it over the head for the time specified in the instructions (Figure 3-2). Be guided by your instructor.

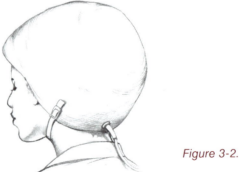

Figure 3-2.

7. When the indicated time is up, work the conditioner through to the ends of the hair.
8. Rinse thoroughly with warm water.

Caution: Do not use hot air from a blow-dryer to facilitate the penetration of the conditioner--the scalp might become irritated. A cool dryer, heating cap, or steamer can be used if necessary to help penetration. NEVER apply heat in any form to a penetrating conditioner BEFORE a chemical service is given. This will open the pores in the scalp and possibly cause irritation when the chemicals are applied.

Instant Conditioners

Instant conditioners coat the hair, giving it body and shine. They flatten raised cuticles, make hair soft and manageable and help to protect the inner structure of the hair shaft from damage by acting as a barrier. Instant conditioners can contain lanolin, cholesterol, moisturizers, sulfonated oil, vegetable oil, proteins, polymers, or some combination of the above.

Procedure for Instant Conditioners

1. Rinse the hair thoroughly.
2. Apply a generous though not excessive amount of instant conditioner.
3. Gently work through the hair to the ends. Comb for even distribution.
4. Leave on for 1 to 5 minutes depending on product chosen.
5. Rinse thoroughly.
6. Detangle with a wide-tooth comb (this will further help to flatten raised cuticles).

TYPES OF CONDITIONERS

Depending on the needs of the client's hair and/or the service requested, protein conditioners, pH balancers, hot oil treatments, or moisturizing conditioners might be necessary.

Protein Conditioners

Protein conditioners are made from partially **hydrolyzing (HI-drol-iz-ing),** or breaking apart, proteins. These can be derived from keratin (the protein that makes up human hair), collagen, or elastin. Other protein conditioners contain animal placentas, panthanol, vegetable extracts, yeast, milk, fish oil or vitamins such as B_6. Conditioners made from animal proteins and keratin are the most effective because they can penetrate into the cortex and repair damage. Penetrating protein conditioners repair damage from chemical services such as lightening or soft curl perming. They improve the way hair looks and feels, bind split ends and improve sheen. The more damaged the hair is, the more conditioner will be able to penetrate. Virgin hair will absorb only small amounts of a protein conditioner.

Protein conditioners also protect the hair from further abuse by coating the cuticle layer. They usually contain **polymers (POL-i-merz),** or long chain molecules, that envelop the hair shaft and keep it strong and protected.

pH Balancers

After a chemical service, your client's hair will still be overly alkaline. A slightly acidic conditioner called a pH balancer will help the hair return more quickly to its pH balance between 4.5 and 5.5. Apply according to manufacturer's directions, leave on 1 to 5 minutes, and rinse.

Hot Oil Treatments

Hot oil treatments are deep penetrating conditioners that are used on hair which is extremely dry or damaged. The application of oil lubricates the hair, softens it, and makes it shiny. It is not the oil itself that repairs the hair, but the protein hydrolysates, polymers, and other ingredients, which are aided in penetration through the heat used with the product.

Procedure

1. Determine the overall condition of the hair and scalp.
2. Shampoo the hair.
3. Part the hair into four sections.
4. Heat the oil to a moderate temperature in hot water.
5. Apply conditioner directly from the tube to hair sections.
6. Massage gently into hair.
7. If the product calls for a plastic cap or other covering, place on the client's head and leave it on the hair for the time specified in the instructions. Be guided by your instructor.
8. Work conditioner through to the ends of the hair.
9. Rinse with warm water.

MOISTURIZERS

Moisturizers are different than conditioners. Most moisturizers specifically formulated for Black hair have glycerine as the main ingredient. They are used for the maintenance of your clients' hair, to make the hair shiny and moist in appearance. Some moisturizers are used to lubricate the scalp. Some manufacturers claim that their moisturizers can *reactivate* curl formation but there is no evidence to support such claims. Moisturizers come in gel, cream, and spray form. Advise clients to use these products sparingly, and not every day, because buildup occurs and becomes difficult to remove through shampooing. Product buildup leads to clogged pores in the scalp, which can eventually lead to diseased hair follicles and hair loss. You may want to emphasize to clients that although moisturizers can make hair more attractive and the scalp moist, they are not a physical necessity except in cases of extreme dryness.

Cream Moisturizers

Cream moisturizer comes in bottle and tube form. It may be used on the hair and scalp. It is applied to damp hair and worked through to the ends with the fingers. Hair is then styled to the desired look.

Gel Moisturizers

Gel moisturizers are packaged in jars or tubes and may be used as a styling aid as well as for giving hair a moist sheen. They are not used on the scalp. Gels can be drying to the scalp so be sure to apply only to the hair shaft. Gel moisturizers are applied by breaking down the product to a liquid form in the hands and working through damp hair to the ends with the fingers. Hair is then shaped into the desired style.

Spray Moisturizers

Spray moisturizers are used primarily to add sheen to a finished style. They are simply sprayed onto the hair after the desired style had been achieved. Many manufacturers of soft curl perms include in their packaging spray moisturizers specifically formulated to go with their products. Always follow the manufacturer's guidelines and be guided by your instructor.

General Moisturizers

There are moisturizing conditioners formulated for use on hair of all races (Figure 3-3). They are formulated to lubricate very dry hair and scalp where little if any natural sebum is present. These conditioners contain ingredients such as silicone derivatives, quaternary ammonium compounds, and oils. They are rinsed off the hair and leave a beneficial, protective film behind that prevents moisture loss. They do not penetrate into the hair shaft.

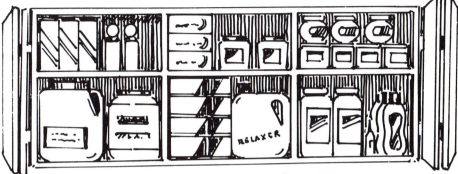

Figure 3-3.

CONDITIONING FOR A SERVICE

What conditioner you use on the hair will depend in part on the state of the hair and whether you are cutting, styling, or chemically servicing it. How you condition your clients' hair will have a tremendous effect on the finished style.

Conditioning for Chemically Processed Hair

When hair has undergone a chemical service and is dry and damaged, it is best to use a penetrating protein conditioner followed by a general moisturizer. If hair is in a very damaged state because of prior processing and a client is requesting a chemical service, a series of penetrating protein conditionings should be given over several salon visits until the hair is in a healthier state. Only then should a new chemical service be given. When hair is slightly damaged you **can** chemically process the hair if you protect it by coating it with conditioner before giving the service.

To keep the processed hair looking shiny, a glycerine-based moisturizer can be applied occasionally by the client at home, and a deep penetrating conditioner given once a week.

Conditioning Before and After a Cut and Style

Virgin hair that is to be cut and styled without the aid of a blow dryer or other thermal appliance should be washed and a light instant conditioner applied and rinsed out before the cut begins. There are also lotions that are designed to be left in the hair during the cut. For conditioning chemically processed hair that is to be cut and styled, see above.

21

Conditioning Hair for Blow-Drying or Thermal Styling

Just before blow-drying or thermal styling a client's hair, be sure to add a styling agent such as styling lotion, mousse or gel. Not only will these products aid in styling the hair, they will also protect the hair from heat damage.

Conditioning for Maintenance

Generally, hair that is coarse and dry should receive an oil based instant conditioning after every shampoo. A protein conditioner will probably be too strong for this hair. Normal hair that is coarse should receive an instant conditioner every couple of weeks. Oily hair that is coarse should get a mild acidic rinse after shampooing. An acid rinse will help to close the cuticle and reduce oiliness. Be sure to thoroughly cleanse the rinse from the hair with cool water. Oily hair of medium texture should also use this rinse. Normal hair of medium texture should use a penetrating protein conditioner once a week. Medium textured hair that is dry should use a deep penetrating conditioner once a week. Soft textured hair that is oily should use the acid rinse. Soft hair that is dry should use a deep penetrating protein conditioner after every shampoo. Soft hair that is normal should use an instant conditioner after each shampoo.

SCALP MANIPULATIONS

Scalp manipulations stimulate the circulation of the blood to the scalp, relax and soothe the nerves, and stimulate the muscles and glands of the scalp. The scalp is made more flexible by massage, and the buildup of moisturizing and conditioning products (when present) is broken down and made easier to remove during shampooing.

Do not give a scalp treatment:

1. If there are abrasions or a scalp disorder present.
2. Immediately before the application of a chemical service.

Procedure

1. Drape the client.
2. Examine the hair and scalp.
3. Shampoo the hair.
4. Part the hair into four sections and apply pomade or massage cream, section by section, until the entire scalp is covered.
5. Begin scalp manipulations (Figures 3-4 through 3-15).

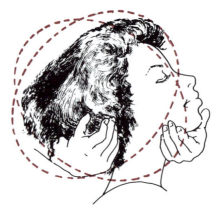

Figure 3-4. RELAXING MOVEMENT. Cup the client's chin in your left hand; place your right hand at the base of his or her skull and rotate the head gently. Reverse the positions of your hands and repeat.

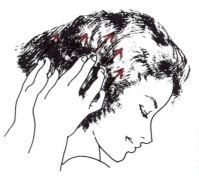

Figure 3-5. SLIDING MOVEMENT. Place your fingertips on each side of the client's head; slide your hands firmly upward, spreading the fingertips until they meet at the top of the head. Repeat four times.

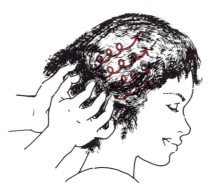

Figure 3-6. SLIDING AND ROTATION MOVEMENT. Same as movement in Figure 3-5 except that after sliding the fingertips one inch, you rotate and move the client's scalp. Repeat four times.

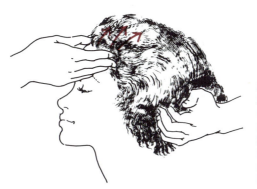

Figure 3-7. FOREHEAD MOVEMENT. Hold the client's head with your left hand. Place stretched thumb and fingers of your right hand on the client's forehead. Move your hand slowly and firmly upward to one inch past the hairline. Repeat four times.

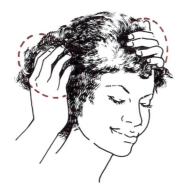

Figure 3-8. SCALP MOVEMENT. Place the palms of your hands firmly against the client's scalp. Lift the scalp in a rotary movement, first with your hands placed above the client's ears, and then with your hands placed at the front and back of his or her neck.

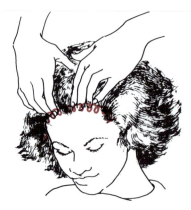

Figure 3-9. HAIRLINE MOVEMENT. Place the fingers of both hands at the client's forehead. Massage around the hairline by lifting and rotating.

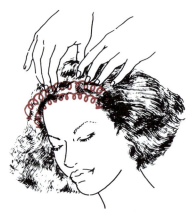

Figure 3-10. FRONT SCALP MOVEMENT. Dropping back one inch, repeat the preceding movement over the entire front and top of the scalp.

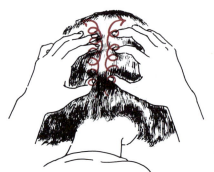

Figure 3-11. BACK SCALP MOVEMENT. Place the fingers of each hand on the sides of the client's head. Starting below the ears, manipulate the scalp with your thumbs, working upward to the crown. Repeat four times. Repeat thumb manipulations, working toward the center back of the head.

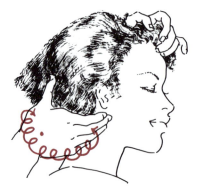

Figure 3-12. EAR-TO-EAR MOVEMENT. Place your left hand on the client's forehead. Massage from the right ear to the left ear along the base of the skull with the heel of your hand, using a rotary movement.

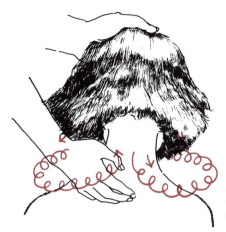

Figure 3-13. BACK MOVEMENT. Place your left hand on the client's forehead and stand to his or her left. Using your right hand, rotate from the base of the client's neck along the shoulder and back across the shoulder blade to the spine. Slide your hand up to the client's spine to the base of the neck. Repeat on the opposite side.

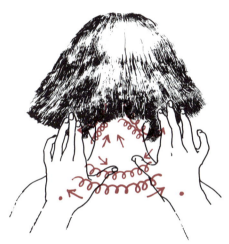

Figure 3-14. SHOULDER MOVEMENT. Place both your palms together at the base of the client's neck. With rotary movements, catch muscles in the palms and massage along the shoulder, and then back again. Then massage from the shoulder to the spine and back again.

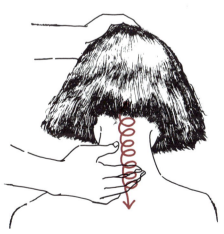

Figure 3-15. SPINE MOVEMENT. Massage from the base of the client's skull down the spine with a rotary movement. Using a firm finger pressure, bring your hand slowly to the base of the client's skull.

RETAILING PRODUCTS FOR MAINTENANCE

After you have completed work on the client's hair, it is very important that you stress the importance of keeping hair in optimum condition between salon visits. This can be done by the client, in part, through the use of a quality conditioner. Your client should be able to buy such a conditioner from the salon in which you will be working. Educate your clients as to the type of conditioner best suited to their hair needs and guide them to buy such a product from the retail counter at the front of the salon. Get to know the product line so you can honestly point out all its merits to your clients. You can do this by talking to a product line representative as well as trying the different products on other stylists in the salon and yourself.

QUESTIONS FOR REVIEW

1. What are the benefits of instant and penetrating conditioners?
2. What is the procedure for a penetrating conditioner?
3. What are three types of moisturizers? What does each do?
4. How should you condition dry, damaged hair that has undergone a chemical service?
5. How are the 12 scalp manipulations done?
6. What is the best way to get to know the product line of conditioners you will be recommending to clients?

Chapter 4   Braiding

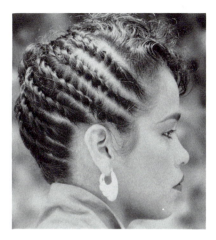

LEARNING OBJECTIVES

After you have mastered this chapter, you will be able to:

1. Give the procedure for plait braiding.
2. Show the procedure for French braiding.
3. Explain how the cornrowing technique differs from the French braiding technique.
4. Give the procedure for the forty-strand braid.
5. List seven tips for braiding.

INTRODUCTION

Braiding has been a popular styling technique throughout history. It has both African and Egyptian origins. Braiding keeps hair smooth and neat, and professional braiding can last longer than more conventional hairstyles. Mastery of this art can make the cosmetologist an asset to any salon servicing Black clients. There are four types of braiding: plait, French, cornrowing, and forty strand.

Plait Braiding

This is the simplest form of braiding. What distinguishes the ***plait braid*** from other braiding techniques is that it is produced from one or more sections of hair (Figure 4-1). The scalp serves as the base, but the plait then leaves the scalp to move freely. This type of braid is most easily done on medium-length to long hair.

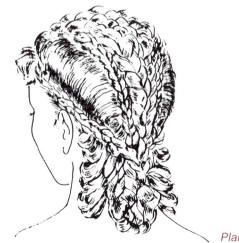

Plait braid

Procedure   Part and section hair in the same manner as for regular French braid.

1. Divide top right section evenly into three strands. Start to braid the hair strands by placing the right side strand under the center strand, and the left side strand under this one. Draw strands tighly. (Fig. 4-2)

2. Pick up ½" (1.25 cm) strand on right side and combine with right side strand. Place this combined strand under the center strand. Pick up ½" (1.25 cm) strand on left side and combine with left side strand. Place this combined strand under center strand. (Fig. 4-3)

3. Continue to pick up hair and braid as above. (Fig. 4-4) Finish braiding at nape, and hold in position with rubber bands.

4. Braid left side of head in the same manner as right side. (Fig. 4-5)

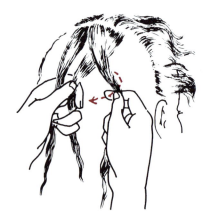
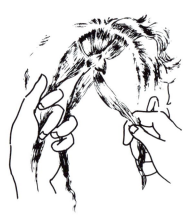

Figure 4-2.   *Figure 4-3.*

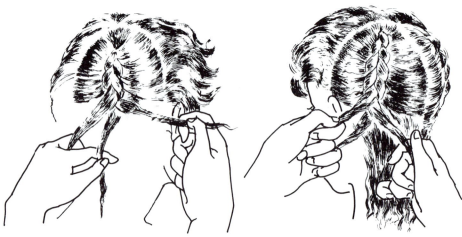

Figure 4-4.   *Figure 4-5.*

FRENCH BRAIDING   **French braiding** involves a close-to-the-head braiding technique and normally consists of one or two large, thick braids lying close to the scalp (Figure 4-6). This type of braiding is especially effective on long hair, but can also be done successfully on medium-length hair. The sections of a French braid overlap on top of one another, with the braid forming on the underside. This gives the top side of the braid a flat appearance.

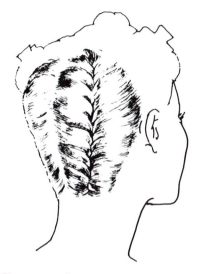

Figure 4-6. French braid

Procedure   1. Part crown section off. Hold out of way with clips or clamps. Back hair: Part hair from center of crown, 1, to nape, 2. (Fig. 4-7)

2. Divide section evenly into three strands. Start to braid by bringing strand 1 (on the left) over strand 2a (in the center) (Fig. 4-8). Draw strands tightly.

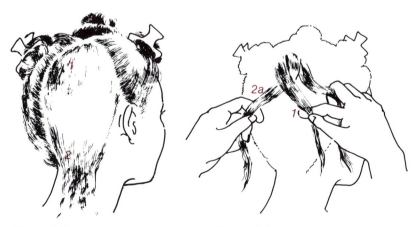

Figure 4-7.   *Figure 4-8.*

3. Pick up another strand from the left, about ½" (1.25 cm) wide, as indicated by 2b (Fig. 4-9). Join strands 2a and 2b. Tighten strands.
4. Bring strand 3 over strand 1 and tighten. (Fig. 4-10) Pick up another strand on the right, about ½" (1.25 cm) wide, and place with strand 1.

> **Note:** *To insure a neat braid with all short hair ends in place, twist each strand toward the right or left with the thumb and index finger.*

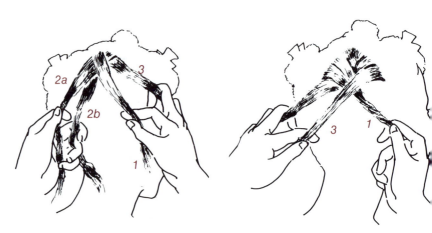

Figure 4-9.

Figure 4-10.

5. Continue to pick up strands and braid (Fig. 4-11), finishing with braiding of hair ends at nape. Fasten with a rubber band or string.
   Braid the left side of the head, following the same procedure. The final regular French braid is illustrated in Fig. 4-12.

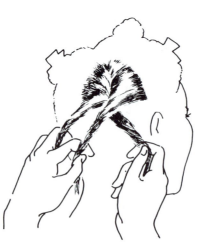

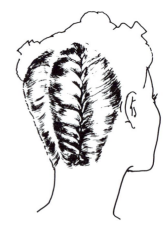

Figure 4-11.

Figure 4-12.

CORNROWING

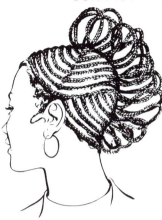

Figure 4-13. Strands are crossed over instead of under in cornrowing.

Cornrowing is also referred to as **inverted braiding.** The procedure is similar to French braiding, except that the strands are crossed *over* instead of *under,* and the picked up strands are added to the strands nearest to the side where you are working (Figure 4-13).

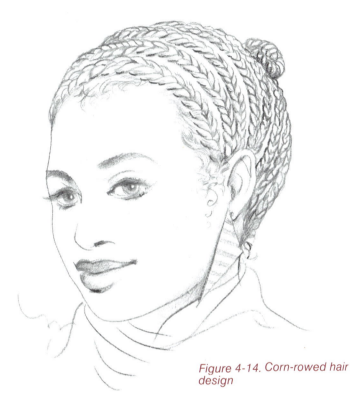

Figure 4-14. Corn-rowed hair design

Cornrow braids are very thin and can be arranged in narrow rows or intricate patterns over the entire head (Figure 4-14).

This type of close-to-the-head braiding is especially effective on short hair.

Follow the procedure for French braiding, paying special attention to the short ends that might become unraveled.

Note: Cornrowed hair must be shampooed with care. Apply a hairnet or stocking to the client's head, making sure the braids are held securely down on the client's scalp. Wet the hair and apply shampoo, using the fingertips to gently massage the scalp and braids, then rinse. Care should be taken to avoid loosening or undoing the braids. Remove the hair net or stocking. Spray the hair with a liquid conditioner. Time according to the manufacturer's instructions. Rinse, towel blot and proceed to condition the scalp or use a spray moisturizer. Cornrowed hair must be shampooed once a week. Techniques for shampooing cornrowed hair can vary. Be guided by your instructor in this matter.

FORTY-STRAND BRAID

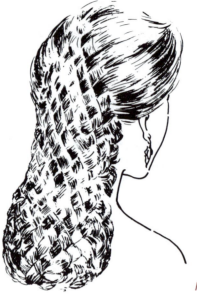

Forty-strand braid

Procedure Pick up a wide section in the center of the lower crown. Divide the section into two parts, then cross the two parts (Figures 4-15 and 4-16).

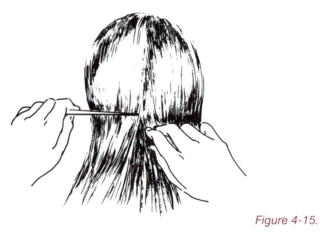

Figure 4-15.

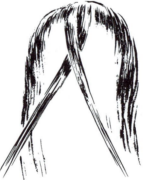

Figure 4-16.

1. Weave the hair from left to right. A third strand is added from the right and crossed over the nearest strand (Figure 4-17).
2. A fourth strand is then lifted from the left side, brought under the strand nearest it, and then brought over the center strand (Figure 4-18).

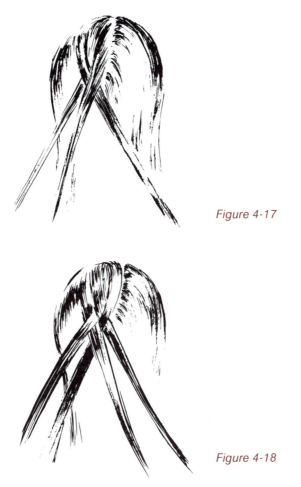

Figure 4-17

Figure 4-18

3. You have now established the two main sections, right and left (Figure 4-19).

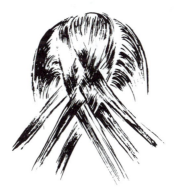

Figure 4-19

4. Continue adding strands, working from right to left, and maintaining the over/under pattern established by the previously woven strands (Figures 4-20 through 4-22). The diamond pattern of the design is now taking shape.

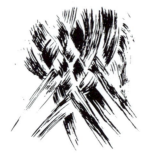

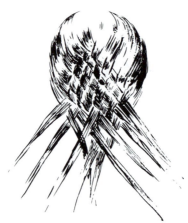

Figure 4-20

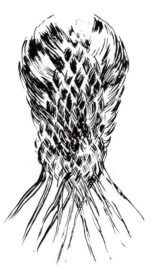

Figure 4-21

Figure 4-22

5. Continue picking up strands of equal diameter to ensure uniform tension and design control. Keep the braided pattern no wider than the head itself. As the braid progresses, there will be fewer strands to work. Those remaining at the bottom may be divided and braided separately (Figure 4-23 through 4-25).

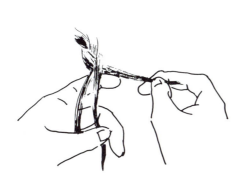

Figure 4-23

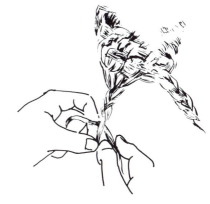

Figure 4-24

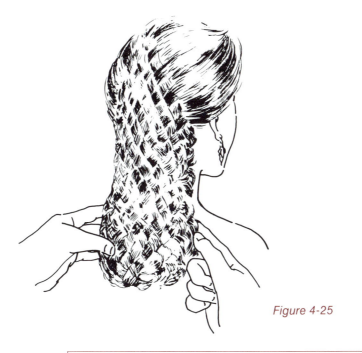

Figure 4-25

Note: A regular three strand braid at the bottom is sufficient, for this will secure the ends and prevent the pattern from unraveling. The ends of the pattern can be secured with fabric-coated elastic bands and tucked under and secured with bobby pins or hair pins to conceal the ends.

BRAIDING TIPS

1. Always be aware of the amount of tension used on the hair while braiding. Too much tension can cause *traction alopecia* (baldness from pulling).
2. Hair that has been chemically treated should be properly conditioned before braiding and should be handled with care.
3. Hair should be shampooed before braiding.
4. If the curl pattern of the hair to be braided is especially tight, a warm pressing comb can be used to loosen the texture before braiding.
5. When wearing a cornrowed style, it is necessary to instruct your client to wash his or her hair weekly.
6. Straight or Caucasian hair is easier to control when wet. Black or excessively curly hair is easier to work with when dry.
7. Braiding is an ideal way to let hair rest between chemical services.
8. Children are well suited for braids, especially in the summer. Use less tension.
9. Small braids are permanent, better for shorter hair, and will create a closer-to-the-head look.
10. Avoid overuse of hair products because they will cause buildup as well as dust to collect on the hair.

QUESTIONS FOR REVIEW

1. What is the procedure for plait braiding?
2. What is the procedure for French braiding?
3. How is the cornrowing technique different from the French braiding technique?
4. What is the procedure for the forty-strand braid?
5. What are seven tips for braiding?

Chapter 5 Hair Shaping

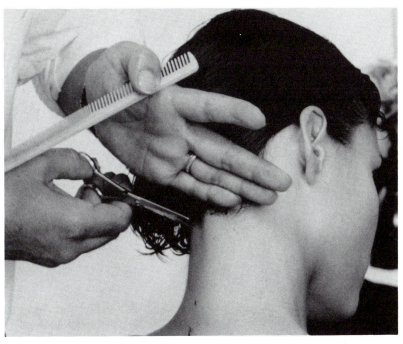

LEARNING OBJECTIVES

After you have mastered this chapter, you will be able to:

1. List two things that must be taken into consideration when shaping Black hair.
2. Demonstrate a five-section parting.
3. List the implements used in Black haircutting.
4. Demonstrate how to hold scissors.
5. Explain why excessively curly hair should be cut dry.
6. Give the procedure for a bob on relaxed hair.
7. Give the procedure for layering Black hair that has not been relaxed.

INTRODUCTION

A good haircut is the foundation for a beautiful hairstyle. As a cosmetologist you must be guided by the client's wishes and by what is best for his or her personality, as well as by your professional expertise. In selecting the proper cut and style, you should evaluate the client's head shape, facial contours, neckline, and hair texture.

SHAPING CONSIDERATIONS

Basic hair shaping is technically the same for all clients. There is the sectioning, selection of the style, cutting with a guideline, and so on. There are, however, two important things to consider when cutting the Black client's hair:

1. Fragility of some hair
2. Curl configuration

SECTIONING

The following information covers the methods for dividing the hair into either four or five sections. In every case, follow your instructor's methods for dry or wet cutting.

Four-Section Parting

Part the hair down the center from the forehead to the nape, and also across the top of the head from ear to ear. Pin up the four sections and leave the nape hair to use as your guide (Figure 5-1).

Five-Section Parting

Part across, starting from behind the ear. Extend the part from ear to ear. Divide the front area into three sections; divide the back area into two sections (Figure 5-2).

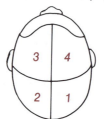

Figure 5-1. Four-section part

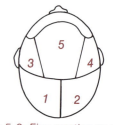

Figure 5-2. Five-section part

> **Caution:** The density and curl pattern of this hair type can make it more difficult to section. Use a large-tooth comb to gently separate the hair at the scalp into four or five sections.

IMPLEMENTS IN BLACK HAIR SHAPING

A cosmetologist will find that the quality of the implements selected and used in haircutting is most important. To do the best work, you should buy and use only superior implements from reliable manufacturers. Improper use will quickly destroy the efficiency of any implement, however finely it might be made in the factory. The following implements are used in Black hair shaping (Figures 5-3a through 5-3g):

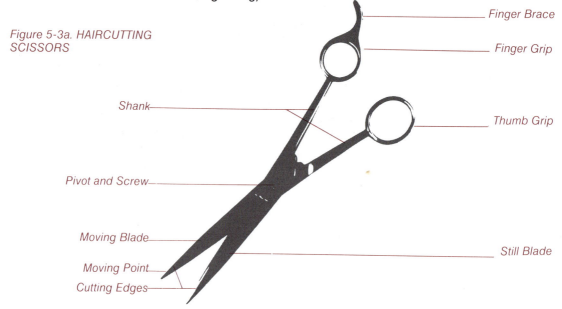

Figure 5-3a. HAIRCUTTING SCISSORS

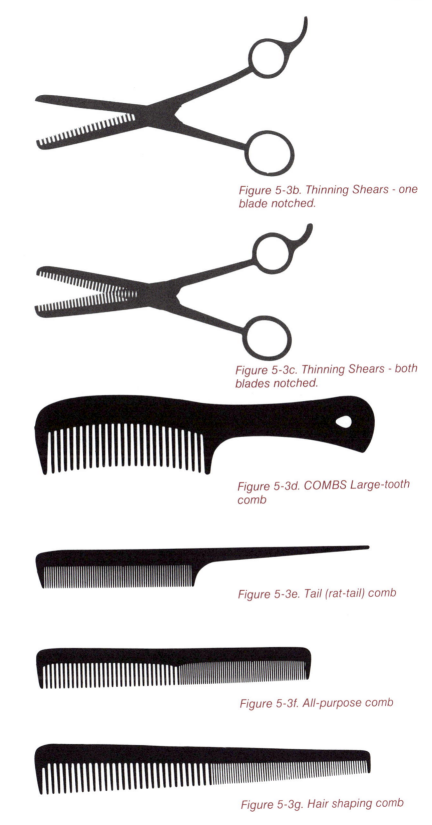

Figure 5-3b. Thinning Shears - one blade notched.

Figure 5-3c. Thinning Shears - both blades notched.

Figure 5-3d. COMBS Large-tooth comb

Figure 5-3e. Tail (rat-tail) comb

Figure 5-3f. All-purpose comb

Figure 5-3g. Hair shaping comb

HOLDING THE IMPLEMENTS Following are the best ways to handle the implements you will be using to cut the hair of your Black client.

Scissors (shears) A pair of scissors is correctly handled by inserting the third (ring) finger into the ring of the still blade and placing the little finger on the finger brace. The thumb is inserted into the ring of the movable blade. The tip of the index finger is braced near the pivot of the scissors for better control (Figure 5-4).

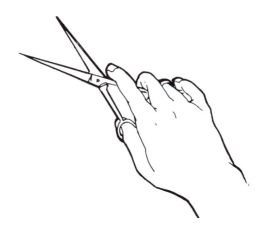

Figure 5-4. How to hold scissors or shears

Comb and Scissors Whenever it is necessary to use a comb during haircutting, close the blades of the scissors, remove your thumb from the ring, and rest the scissors in the palm of your hand. Hold the scissors securely with your ring finger (Figure 5-5).

Note: When combing hair, hold the comb and scissors in the same hand. When cutting hair, hold the comb in the hand that is holding the subsection. To speed hair shaping, do not lay down the comb or scissors.

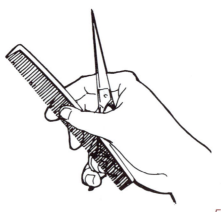

Figure 5-5. How to hold comb and scissors simultaneously

Thinning Shears

Excess bulk is removed from the hair by using thinning shears (Figure 5-6). These shears are similar to scissors except that they have one or both blades notched or serrated. The single notched edge cuts more hair. Which one is used depends on the preference of the cosmetologist. The notches help control the amount of hair that is removed. Both thinning shears and scissors are held the same way.

> **Note:** Razors are seldom used in Black hair shaping except when needed for cleaning the nape area at the finish of certain cuts. Be guided by your instructor on the use of razors in Black haircutting.

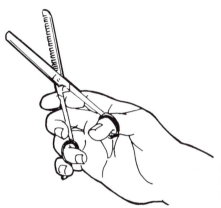

Figure 5-6. Shears are similar to scissors except one or both blades are notched and serrated.

HAIRCUTTING TECHNIQUES

On clients with excessively curly hair, it is better to cut the hair while dry, to take the curl configuration into account when defining the shape, and to avoid an uneven line.

Dry shaping is done before the hair is shampooed, unless the hair is coated with oil or is excessively dirty. In that case, shampoo first, allow the hair to dry naturally or under lamps, avoid relaxing the curl, and proceed with the shaping.

Wet shaping is done directly after shampooing. Hair that has been chemically relaxed or has received a soft curl should be conditioned prior to sectioning. This will make the hair softer and less likely to tangle.

CUTTING CHEMICALLY OR PHYSICALLY RELAXED HAIR

The following is a basic bob cut for the Black client with chemically or physically relaxed hair.

1. Part the hair into four sections (Figure 5-7).
2. Blunt cut a guideline subsection of nape hair using zero elevation (Figure 5-8).
3. Bring down a subsection of hair, parting off hair from the midsection of ears at either side of the head (Figure 5-9). Cut with zero elevation, using the established guideline.
4. Complete the back, remembering to cut with zero elevation and using the established guideline. Avoid using tension throughout the cut.

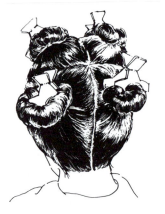

5. Move to the left side of the head and bring down a thin subsection of hair over the ear (Figure 5-10).
6. Bring hair from back to side, cutting a side guideline to match the back guideline (Figure 5-11).
7. Continue to bring the subsections down, cutting to match the established side guideline.
8. Repeat steps 5 through 7 on the right side of the head.

Figure 5-7.

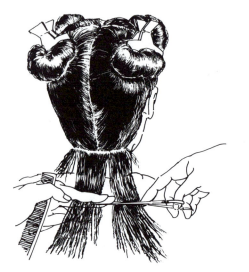

Figure 5-8.

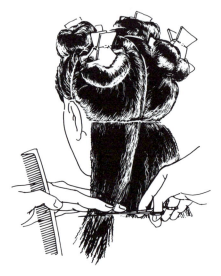

Figure 5-9.

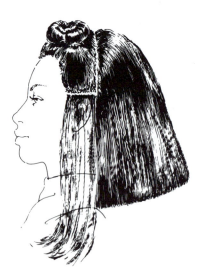

Figure 5-10.

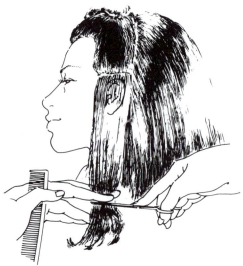

Figure 5-11.

CUTTING VIRGIN (OR NATURAL) HAIR

The steps outlined here represent a basic method of cutting Black hair that has not received a chemical service and is therefore *virgin.* The result of the procedure will be an Afro.

Preparation

1. Drape and prepare the client.
2. Shampoo the hair and dry thoroughly.
3. Lightly apply a conditioning product to the scalp and hair to replace lost oil.

Procedure

1. Using a wide-tooth comb or pick, comb the hair upward and slightly forward, making it as long as possible. Start at the crown and continue until all hair has been distributed evenly around the head. Combing in a circular pattern will usually help avoid splits.
2. Begin the cut by tapering the sides, cutting in the direction that the hair will be combed.
3. Taper the back part of the head to blend with the sides.
4. Trim the extreme hair ends of the crown and top areas to the desired length.
5. For an off-the-face hairstyle, comb the hair up and backward. For forward movement, comb the hair up and forward.
6. Blend the side hair with the top, crown, and back hair.
7. Outline the hairstyle at the sides, around the ears and in the nape area, using either scissors or a clipper.
8. Give a finishing touch. Fluff the hair slightly with a pick, whenever needed. Spray hair lightly to give it a natural, lustrous sheen.

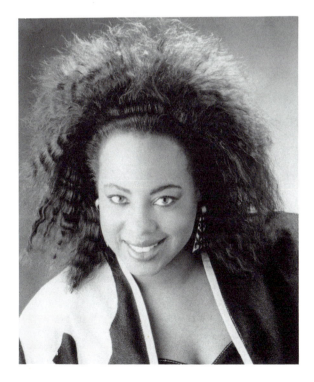

LAYERED LOOKS FOR BLACK HAIR

The following two cuts are basic ones that Black clients are likely to ask for: relaxed and layered and natural and layered.

Relaxed and Layered

This layered look is for the Black client whose hair has been chemically relaxed.

Procedure

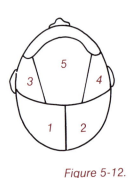

Figure 5-12.

1. Divide the hair into five sections (Figure 5-12).
2. Bring down a 1-inch subsection from the left side of the head, over the ear (Figure 5-13).
3. Bring down a second 1-inch subsection. Hold at a 45-degree angle above the first subsection and cut to establish a guideline (Figure 5-14).
4. Bring down another 1/2-inch section and cut to match the guideline (Figure 5-15).
5. Repeat steps 2 through 4 on the opposite side of the head.
6. Make a parting over the ear and down into the nape. Overdirect the subsection forward to establish a guideline for the back of the head (Figure 5-16).

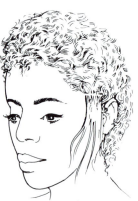

Figure 5-13.

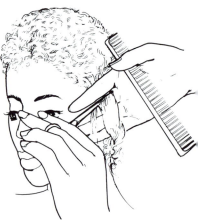

Figure 5-14.

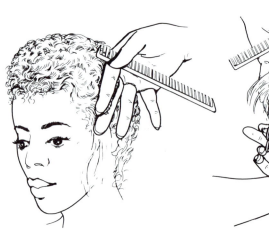

Figure 5-15.

Figure 5-16.

7. Repeat step 6 on the opposite side of the head.

8. Blend the rest of the hair on either side of the head. Hold the subsection at a 45-degree angle and cut even with the guideline established in step 6 (Figure 5-17).

9. Comb the front section of the hair back to the crown at a 180-degree angle and cut to establish a guideline for length (Figure 5-18).

10. Pick up a subsection at the top of the head, combing as shown toward the crown. Begin layering by cutting hair at a 45-degree angle short to long, to blend top to back. Using portions of all three guidelines, layer toward the back of the head, holding the subsections at a 90-degree angle (Figure 5-19).

11. Comb sides into the top guideline and cut for blend.

12. Double-check the blend in the back by combing into the side and top guidelines.

13. Finish the sides by establishing a length to adapt to the client's facial features and his or her wishes.

14. The haircut may be thermal styled or set to finish (Figure 5-20).

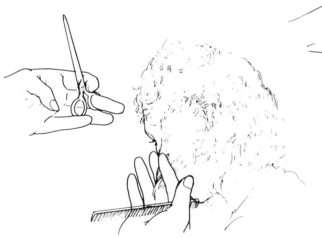

Figure 5-17.

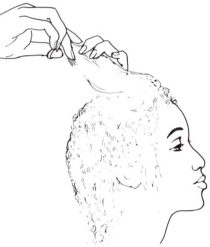

Figure 5-18.

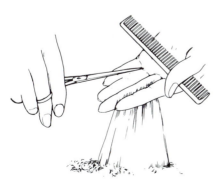

Figure 5-19.

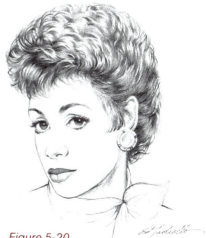

Figure 5-20.

Natural and Layered

This cut is for the Black client whose hair has not been chemically relaxed and is worn either naturally or in a soft curl perm.

Procedure

1. Divide the hair into five sections (Figure 5-21).

2. Bring down and cut a thin subsection of hair to establish a guideline, holding the subsection close to the client's face and cutting across the bridge of the nose (Figure 5-22).

3. Begin cutting vertical subsections in the top section, moving out to the edges of the section and holding subsections at a 90-degree angle (Figure 5-23).

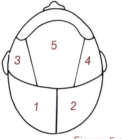

Figure 5-21.

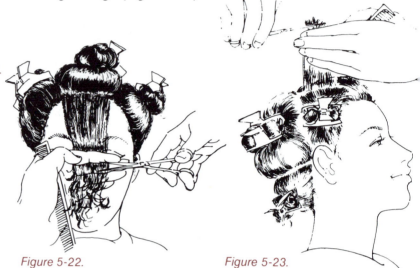

Figure 5-22.   Figure 5-23.

4. Move to a section at the side of the head and establish a guideline by directing a thin subsection from the hairline toward the front of the head and cutting to match the length of the front section (Figure 5-24).

5. Continue to cut vertical subsections held at a 90-degree angle, moving back toward the ear, until the entire section is cut (Figure 5-25).

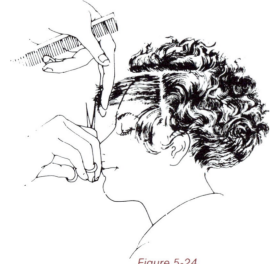

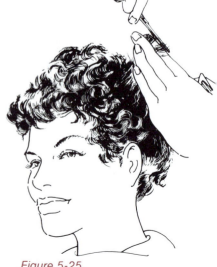

Figure 5-24.   Figure 5-25.

6. Repeat steps 4 and 5 on the side section at the opposite side of the head.
7. At the crown of the head, hold the hair out at a 90-degree angle and cut, using previously cut subsections as your guide (Figure 5-26).

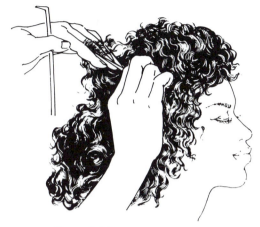

Figure 5-26.

8. Continue to cut horizontal subsections, held at a 90-degree angle, down the back of the head (Figure 5-27).
9. Finish the cut by blending hair around the perimeter of the style; holding the scissors diagonally and subsections close to the head (Figure 5-28).

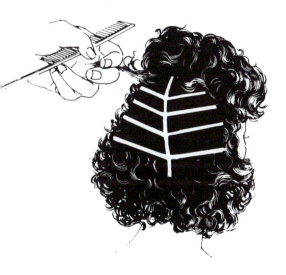

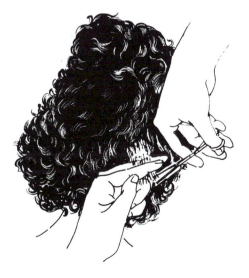

Figure 5-27.   *Figure 5-28*

1. What are two things to be taken into consideration when cutting Black hair?

2. How do you do a five-section parting?

3. What are the implements used in Black haircutting?

4. How is a pair of scissors held?

5. Why should excessively curly hair be cut dry?

6. What is the procedure for a bob on relaxed hair?

7. What is the procedure for layering Black hair that has not been relaxed?

Chapter 6 Hairstyling

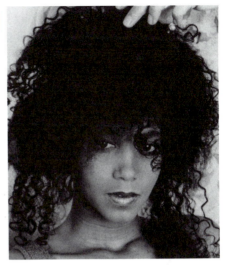

LEARNING OBJECTIVES

After you have mastered this chapter, you will be able to:

1. Describe the roller set for the upsweep style.
2. Name four rules for comb-out.
3. Demonstrate the procedure for hair extensions.
4. Show the proper way to brush an extension.

INTRODUCTION

Beautiful styles for Black hair can be successfully achieved with roller sets or hair extensions. Best results are usually seen when the hair has been relaxed by either thermal or chemical means before the styling begins.

ROLLER SETS

There is no difference between roller setting relaxed Black hair and Caucasian hair; the same procedures and principles apply. It should be noted, however, that when working with Black hair, proper tension must be maintained during the set to ensure that the hair at the base remains straight during the drying process.

Following are some basic styles for Black hair that require a roller set.

Upsweep

This classic style will serve your client well in the office as well as for an evening out (Figure 6-1).

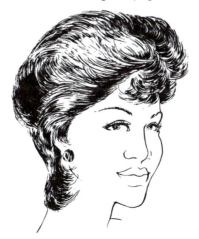

Figure 6-1. Upseep hairstyle

Procedure

1. Divide the hair into five sections (Figure 6-2).
2. Starting from above the right ear, take 1 1/2-inch sections and place on rollers in an on-base direction, moving toward the outer edge of the left eyebrow (Figure 6-3).
3. Starting from above the left ear, take 1 1/2-inch sections and place on rollers in an on-base direction moving up toward the eyebrow (Figure 6-4).
4. At the left side of the crown, direct rollers in an off-base direction moving downward, again using 1 1/2-inch sections (Figure 6-5).
5. At the right side of the crown, roll 1 1/2-inch sections in an off-base direction moving upward (Figure 6-5).
6. At the nape area, roll 1 1/2-inch sections in an on-base direction, moving from right to left to blend with an upsweep effect on the side (Figure 6-5).
7. Place the client under the dryer for approximately 45 minutes or until the hair is completely dry.

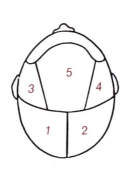

Figure 6-2. Five-section part

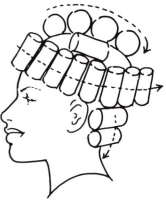

Figure 6-3.

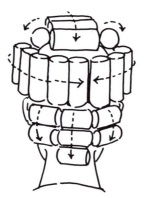

Figure 6-4.

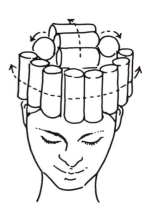

Figure 6-5.

Pageboy   This is a sleek look that many clients will request (Figure 6-6).

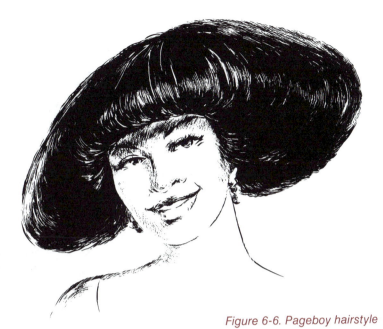

Figure 6-6. Pageboy hairstyle

Procedure   1. Comb the hair into the desired style with no visible parts or separations in the crown or bang areas.

2. Starting at the crown area, drag hair about 3 inches or to the occipital bone and place on rollers in an off-base position, rolling downward. Place rollers side by side moving around both sides of the head (Figure 6-7). Make two or three tiers of rollers depending on the length of the hair.

3. At the bang area two to three rollers, rolled downward, should be sufficient (Figure 6-8).

4. Place the client under the dryer for approximately 45 minutes.

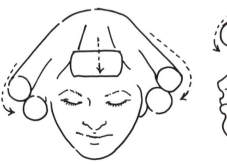

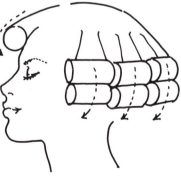

Figure 6-7.

Figure 6-8.

Long and Curly Look   A soft, romantic, yet basic style for clients with longer hair (Figure 6-9).

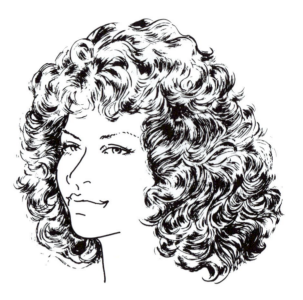

Figure 6-9. Long and curly look

Procedure

1. At the front of the head make a zigzag part.
2. Take 1-inch sections of hair and place curlers in an on-base position, rolling downward (Figure 6-10). Move down from the parting to the top of the ears.
3. At the crown of the head, place three curlers, graduating in size from small to large, in an off-base position moving backward (Figure 6-11).
4. Move to the back of the head. At the crown place medium-sized rollers in an on-base position, rolled to the left. Place a second row of curlers directly underneath the first, at ear level, and roll to the right (Figure 6-11).
5. Directly beneath the second row of curlers, place smaller curlers in an on-base position, moving downward to the nape (Figure 6-12).

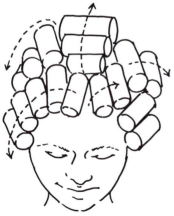

Figure 6-10.

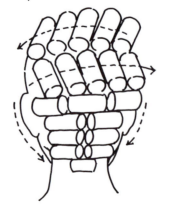

Figure 6-11.

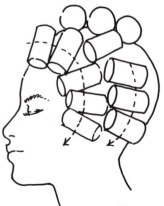

Figure 6-12.

Short and Layered   This is a popular style that most clients will find attractive and easy to care for (Figure 6-13).

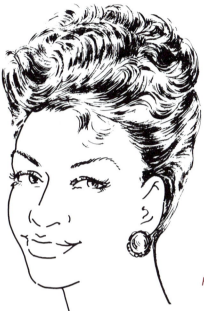

Figure 6-13. Short and layered look

Procedure
1. Divide the hair into five sections.
2. Roll the middle section back to the crown using 1-inch sections (Figure 6-14).
3. At the left temple, roll the remaining two top sections in an on-base position, rolling back to the crown (Figure 6-15).
4. Repeat step 4 at the right temple.
5. Move to the back of the head. From the crown to the occipital bone place curlers on-base, rolling downward. As you get closer to the nape, use smaller curlers (Figure 6-16).

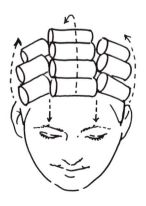

Figure 6-14.

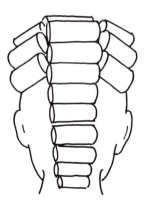

Figure 6-15.

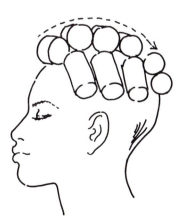

Figure 6-16.

COMB-OUT   The comb-out procedure is very important to the final look of the style you have created. The following rules will help you to give your client the smart style you intended.

1. Follow the lines of the design with a brush to relax curls and blend shape.
2. Dry mold the style by retracing the lines of the style with a comb.
3. Back brushing or back combing is optional. It serves to give you control of the style and to give the style height and form. When doing this step, remember to connect all lines so that the shapes blend well. For higher volume, the hair is held straight up and back combed from underneath. For less volume in areas such as the nape, hold the hair flat to the head and back comb on top.
4. Complete the procedure by smoothing over the back combing with a brush or comb and defining the lines of the hair for various effects.
5. Use hair accessories or artistic detailing to enhance the appearance or effect of an overall design.

HAIR EXTENSIONS   Hair extensions are a good way to make your client's hair longer, fuller, or both. This service is popular with men and women and is very helpful to the client whose hair is thinning or who suffers a certain degree of baldness. Real or synthetic hair may be used in this procedure with looks that can range from intricate braids to a wild and brightly colored add-on for special effect.

Implements and Materials

Vent brush
Clips
Extensions or wefts
Needles
Adhesive

Wide-tooth comb
Extension scissors
Thread
Rubber bands

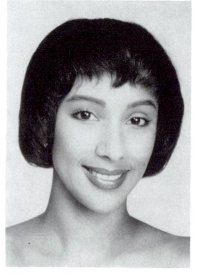

Before addition of hair extension

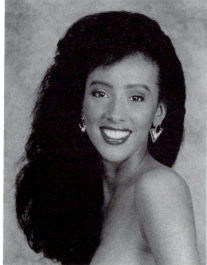

After addition of hair extension

Procedure

1. Decide on the hairstyle to be created, bearing in mind the client's life-style, facial features, and desire.

2. Choose the extensions that most closely match the color and texture desired by the client.

3. If a service such as coloring or permanent waving is to be performed on the client, do it at this point, before extensions are added. Both services may be performed on the extensions themselves before they are added to the client's hair. This is done by attaching the extensions to a mannequin made especially for use with hair extensions, and then performing the chemical service. Consult the manufacturer's directions and your instructor to make sure your brand of extension can withstand a chemical service.

4. Part the hair horizontally from ear to ear (Figure 6-17). Pull the hair up above the part, out of the way, and clip.

5. Split the hair below the part into four separate sections and clip each one at the bottom (Figure 6-18).

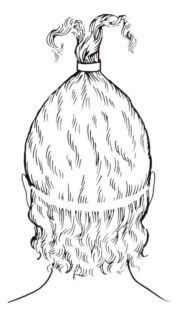

Figure 6-17.

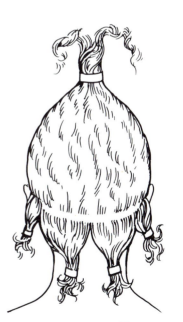

Figure 6-18.

6. Cornrow a braid from the left end of the part to the center and then from the right end of the part to the center (Figure 6-19).

7. Loosely braid the end of each cornrow, then tuck the end snugly underneath the row. An alternative method to this step is to clip together the right and left cornrows where they meet in the middle of the part and let the remaining hair hang down in a ponytail that is secured at the end (Figure 6-20).

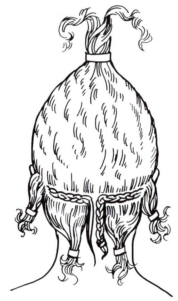

Figure 6-19.

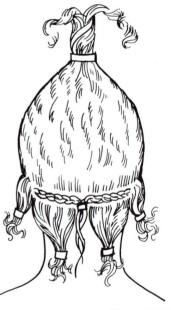

Figure 6-20.

8. With the thick cotton thread and needle made especially for use with extensions, sew the tucked-under end of each cornrow to the cornrows, making sure to knot the thread when you are done. Be careful not to braid the client's hair too tightly because it will be uncomfortable and could cause hair loss. Check to make sure the skin is not pulled away from the scalp when the braid is finished. When using synthetic extensions, a heating clamp is sometimes applied to fuse the natural hair to the extension. Be guided by the manufacturer's directions and your instructor.

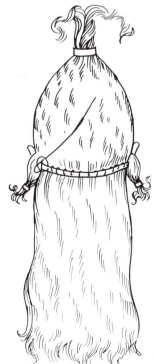

9. Take the hair extension and measure by holding it against the cornrowed part. If it is too long, cut accordingly, using scissors specifically made for hair extensions (Figure 6-21).

10. Double thread the needle and sew a knot to the right end of the edging of the extension (Figure 6-22).

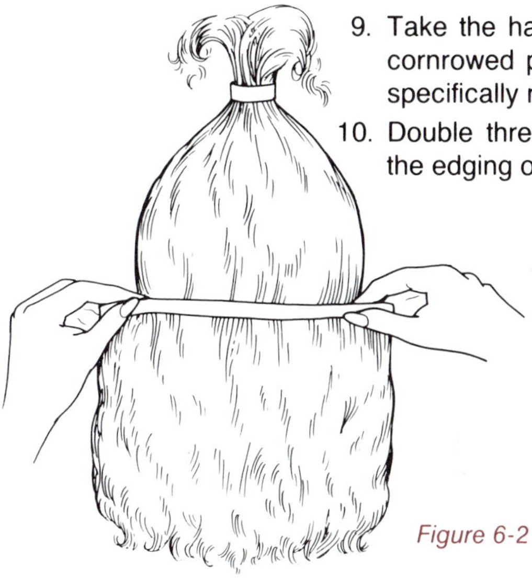

Figure 6-21.

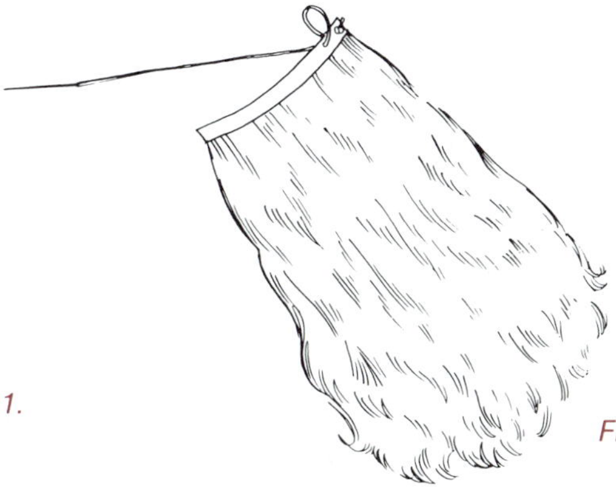

Figure 6-22.

11. Place the extension against the cornrows. Begin to sew the extension to the part, starting from the right-hand side.

12. Bring the needle behind and under the cornrow, then up around and through the edging of the extension (Figure 6-23).

13. Continue to sew in this manner until the extension is attached to the entire length of the part (Figure 6-24). When you get to the left end of the edging, cut the end of the thread and make a double knot. Stitches along the extension should be evenly placed and tight.

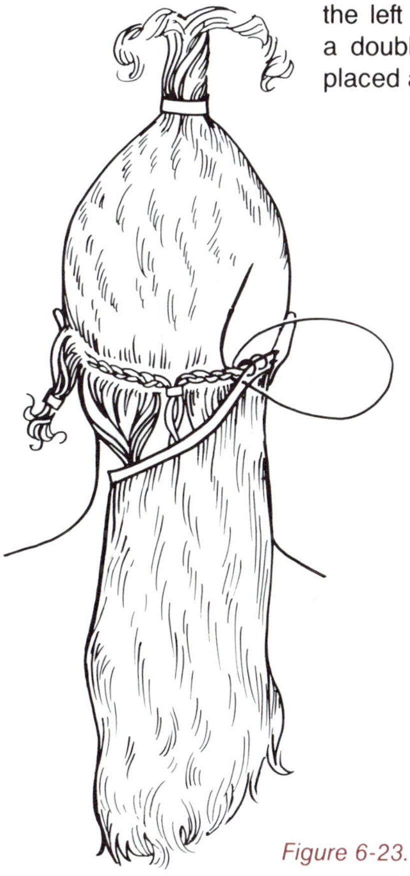

Figure 6-23.

Figure 6-24.

14. Continue to make parts and attach extensions until the desired style is achieved. Always make sure there is enough natural hair to cover the places where the extension is attached to the part. Several types of adhesives, both temporary and extended hold, are available to glue the extensions directly to the hair. Follow the manufacturer's directions and your instructor before using these products.

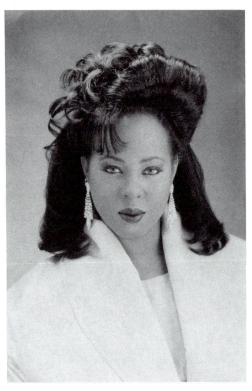

STYLING AND AFTER-CARE OF EXTENSIONS

Most types of hair extensions, both synthetic and natural, can be blown dry, set, crimped, or curled with hot curlers or a curling iron. Curled extensions should be picked not brushed, and when brushing other types of extensions, they should be held close to the point of attachment and brushed downward from there.

Clients should be carefully instructed as to how to properly care for their extensions once the style has been finished. Shampoos and conditioners especially formulated for use with extensions should be available to the client from the retail counter in the salon.

QUESTIONS FOR REVIEW

1. How is the roller set for the upsweep done?
2. What are four rules for comb-out?
3. What is the procedure for hair extensions?
4. How should an extension be brushed?

Chapter 7   Chemical Hair Relaxing

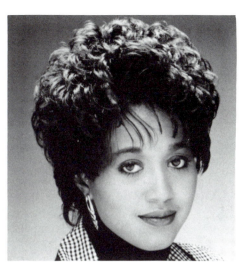

LEARNING OBJECTIVES

After you have mastered this chapter, you will be able to:

1. Explain the chemical actions of sodium hydroxide and neutralizer on the hair.
2. Give the three basic relaxing steps.
3. Explain the procedure for a relaxer test.
4. List the steps in the procedure for relaxing with sodium hydroxide.
5. Explain how the conditioner filler works.
6. Give the procedure for the sodium hydroxide retouch.
7. Explain how ammonium thioglycolate differs from sodium hydroxide in its effect on curly hair.
8. Name other types of relaxer.
9. List 18 safety precautions to follow in chemical relaxing.

INTRODUCTION

Chemical hair relaxing is the process of permanently rearranging the basic structure of excessively curly hair so that it takes on a straighter form. When done professionally, it leaves the hair manageable and in good condition so that it can be set or styled in many ways.

CHEMICAL HAIR RELAXING PRODUCTS

The basic products that are used in chemical hair relaxing are a **chemical hair relaxer**, a **neutralizer** (also known as neutralizing shampoo or stabilizer), and a **petroleum cream**, which is used as a protective base for the client's scalp during a sodium hydroxide chemical relaxing process.

Chemical Hair Relaxers

The two general types of hair relaxers are **sodium hydroxide**, which does not allow for pre-shampooing, and **ammonium thioglycolate**, which does allow for pre-shampooing if needed.

Sodium hydroxide. This has both a softening and a swelling action on hair fibers. As the relaxer cream penetrates in the cortical layer, the cross bonds (sulfur and hydrogen) are broken. The action of the comb, the brush, or the hands in smoothing the hair and distributing the chemical straightens the softened hair.

Manufacturers vary the sodium hydroxide content of the solution from 5 to 10 percent and the pH factor from 10 to higher. In general, the more sodium hydroxide used and the higher the pH, the quicker the chemical reaction will take place on the hair, and the greater the danger of hair damage.

Ammonium thioglycolate (thio type relaxer). Although ammonium thioglycolate is less dramatic in its action than sodium hydroxide, it softens and relaxes excessively curly hair in somewhat the same manner.

Neutralizer

The neutralizer is also called a stabilizer or fixative. It stops the action of any chemical relaxer that remains in the hair after rinsing. At the same time, the neutralizer reforms the cystine (sulfur) cross bonds in their new position and rehardens the hair.

> *Caution:* Because of the high alkaline content of sodium hydroxide, great care must be exercised in its use.

Protective Base for Sodium Hydroxide

The protective base is a petroleum cream that is designed to protect the client's skin and scalp during the sodium hydroxide chemical relaxing. This protective base is also important during a chemical relaxing retouch. It is applied to protect the hair that had been relaxed previously and to prevent over-processing and hair breakage.

The petroleum cream has a lighter consistency than petroleum jelly and is formulated to melt at body temperature. The melting process assures the complete coverage of the scalp and other protected areas with a thin, oily coating. This helps to prevent burning and/or irritation of the scalp and skin. Previously treated hair should be protected with cream conditioner during the straightening process.

BASIC RELAXING STEPS

Chemical hair relaxing involves three basic steps: **Processing, neutralizing**, and **conditioning**.

Processing

As soon as the relaxer is applied, the hair begins to soften so that the chemical can penetrate to loosen and relax the natural curl.

Neutralizing

When the hair has been sufficiently processed, the chemical relaxer is thoroughly rinsed with warm water, followed by either a built-in shampoo neutralizer or a prescribed shampoo and neutralizer.

Conditioning

Depending on the client's needs, the conditioner may be part of a series of hair treatments, or it may be applied to the hair before or after the relaxing treatment.

Caution: Excessively curly hair that is damaged due to thermal comb or thermal iron treatments, tinting, or lightening should receive conditioning treatments to give strength and body to the damaged hair to protect it against breakage. Hair treated with metallic dyes must not be given a hair relaxing treatment; to do so would damage or destroy the hair. It is not advisable to use chemical relaxers on hair that has been lightened (bleached).

Recommended Strength of Relaxer

The strength of the relaxer used is determined by the strand test. The following guidelines can help in determining what strength of relaxer to use for the test.

1. Fine, tinted, or lightened hair: Use mild relaxer.
2. Normal, medium-textured virgin hair: Use regular relaxer.
3. Coarse, virgin hair: Use strong or super relaxer.

HAIR ANALYSIS

It is essential that the cosmetologist has a working knowledge of human hair, especially when giving a relaxing treatment. Recognition of the qualities of hair is achieved by means of a visible inspection, feel, and special tests. Before attempting to give a relaxing treatment to Black hair, the cosmetologist must judge its texture, porosity, elasticity, and the extent, if any, of damage to the hair and scalp.

Porosity

It is very important to determine hair porosity before giving a chemical service. Knowing hair porosity will help you to determine the strength of the relaxer and the amount of processing time needed. The more porous the hair, the more readily it will absorb chemicals.

To test for porosity: lift the hair from the scalp with one hand and push the hair strands downward toward the scalp with the other hand. If the hair bunches up as if teased, it is very porous. If the hair bunches up somewhat, it is normal. If the hair bunches little or not at all, then it is resistant (Figure 7-1).

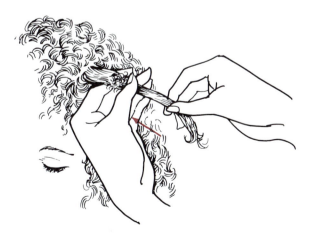

Figure 7.-1. Porosity test

Texture Hair texture refers to the diameter of the individual hair and its degree of fineness or coarseness. The texture and porosity are judged together in determining the processing time. Although the porosity is the more important of the two, texture has an important part in estimating processing time. Fine hair with a small diameter will be saturated with chemicals more quickly than hair with a large diameter, if both are equal in porosity (Figure 7-2).

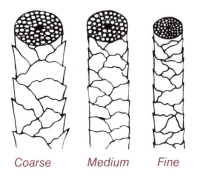

Coarse   *Medium*   *Fine*

Figure 7-2. Hair textures

Variations in hair texture are due to the diameter of the hair shaft, either coarse, medium or fine; the feel of the hair, whether harsh, soft or normal.

Elasticity Hair elasticity is a very important factor when giving a chemical service. Elasticity is the ability of the hair to stretch and contract. All hair is elastic, but its elasticity ranges from very good to poor. When dry, hair should have the ability to stretch 20 percent of its length and return, and 40 percent of its length when wet.

To test the elasticity of the hair, select a hair and hold it between the index finger and thumb of both hands. Gently pull the hair and note its elasticity. If it stretches and returns the correct amount, elasticity is good. If it breaks or stretches, elasticity is poor (Figure 7-3). Poor elasticity is the first clue that there have been too many chemical applications (color, bleaching, previous relaxing, and so on).

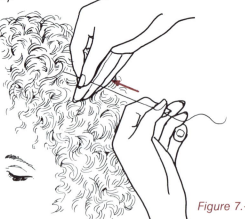

Figure 7.-3. Elasticity test

Elasticity can also be tested by various mechanical devices. Follow the manufacturer's directions for procedure and determining results.

Hair Density   Hair density is the amount of hair per square inch of the scalp. It has nothing to do with the hair's texture. Density determines the amount of the product used and the size of the partings made when applying relaxer.

Scalp Examination   Before beginning the relaxing service, inspect the scalp carefully for eruptions, scratches, or abrasions. To obtain a clear view of the scalp, part the hair into 1/2-inch sections (Figure 7-4). Parting may be done with the index and middle fingers or with the handle of a rattail comb. In either case, the cosmetologist must exercise caution not to scratch the scalp. Such scratches can become infected when irritated by the chemicals in the relaxer.

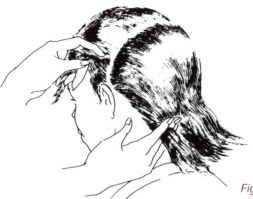

Figure 7.-4. Examining the scalp

> ***Caution:*** If scalp eruptions or abrasions are present, do not apply the chemical hair relaxer until the scalp is in a healthy condition.

Relaxer Test   After assessing the condition of the hair, you are ready to give a **relaxer test.** Applying relaxer to a subsection will indicate its effect on the hair. Take a small section of hair and place it over a piece of aluminum foil (Figure 7-5), as close to the scalp as possible. Apply

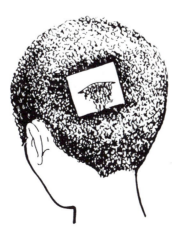

Figure 7.-5. Relaxer strand test

relaxer to the subsection in the same manner you will apply it to the entire head. Process the subsection until it is sufficiently relaxed, checking the strand every 3 to 5 minutes. Make careful note of the timing, the smoothing required, and the hair strength. Shampoo the relaxer from the subsection, towel dry, and cover with protective cream to avoid damage during the relaxing process.

The area selected for the relaxer test should be either the crown or another area where the hair is resistant.

RELAXING PROCESS WITH SODIUM HYDROXIDE

You are now ready to relax the hair. The process outlined here is based primarily on products containing sodium hydroxide. For this or any other product, follow the manufacturer's instructions and be guided by your instructor. This process is for **virgin hair** (hair that has not received prior relaxing or other chemical services). The relaxing product can be applied with a brush, comb, or the fingers.

Equipment, Implements, and Materials Needed

Chemical relaxer	Neutralizer or neutralizing shampoo
Shampoo and finishing rinse	Shampoo cape
Protective base	Conditioner filler
Gloves	Towels
Rollers or blow-dryer and curling iron	Spatula
Timer	Applicator comb or brush
Plastic bowl	Conditioner
Sanitary cotton	Neck strip
Plastic clips	End papers
Setting lotion	Client record card
Brushes and combs for styling	

Preparation

1. Select and arrange the required equipment, implements, and materials.
2. Wash and sanitize your hands.
3. Seat the client comfortably; remove earrings and neck jewelry
4. Adjust the towel and shampoo cape around the client's neck
5. Examine and evaluate the scalp and hair.
6. Give a relaxer test and check the results. Record on a clien card.
7. **Do not** shampoo the hair. (Hair ends may be trimmed after the relaxer is applied.)
8. Have the client sign a release card.

Procedure

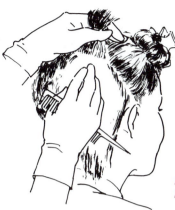

1. Apply a protective base to shield the scalp from the chemicals in the relaxer. To apply, part the hair in four or five distinct sections. Then subdivide each section into 1/2-inch to 1-inch partings to allow for thorough coverage (Figure 7-6).

Figure 7.-6. Applying protective base

2. Divide the hair into four or five sections as recommended by your instructor. Use off-center partings to prevent lasting visible impressions (Figure 7-7). Then subdivide each section.

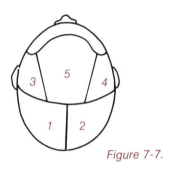

Figure 7-7.

3. Apply the relaxer starting 1/2 to 1 inch from the scalp and spread to within 1/2 inch of the hair ends (Figure 7-8).

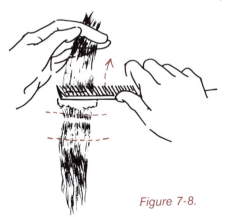

Figure 7-8.

Caution: To protect your hands always wear gloves when applying relaxer.

4. Apply relaxer to each subsection, first to the top side, then the underside (Figures 7-9 and 7-10). After completing each section, gently lay it up out of the way (Figure 7-11). Continue the same process through the remaining three or four sections. The relaxer is applied last to the scalp area and hair ends because less processing time is needed in those places. The client's body heat will speed up the processing action at the scalp, and the hair is more porous at the ends so that these two places process more quickly than other areas.

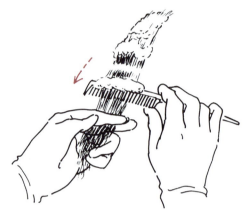

Figure 7.-9. Applying relaxer on top of strand

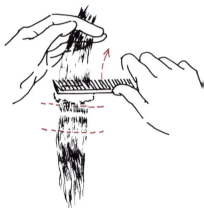

Figure 7.-10. Applying relaxer underneath strand

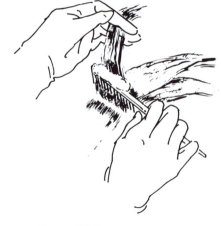

Figure 7-11.

Rinsing Out Relaxer   When the hair has been sufficiently relaxed, rapidly and thoroughly rinse out the relaxer. The water must be warm, not hot. If the water is too hot, it can burn the client and cause discomfort because of the very sensitive condition of the scalp. If the water is too cold, it will not stop the processing. The direct force of the rinse water should be used to remove the relaxer and avoid tangling the hair. Part the hair with the fingers to make sure no traces of the relaxer remain. Relaxer left on the hair continues its chemical action. The stream of water should be directed from the scalp to the hair ends (Figure 7-12).

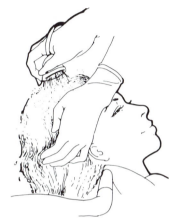

Figure 7.-12. Rinsing out relaxer

Caution: Do not get relaxer or rinse water into the eyes or on unprotected skin. If either gets into the client's eyes, wash it out immediately with large quantities of water and take the client to a doctor without delay. Continue wearing protective gloves until all relaxer has been removed. It is recommended that you blot hair with a towel or cotton.

SHAMPOOING/ NEUTRALIZING AND CONDITIONING   The final steps in the relaxing process are shampooing/neutralizing and conditioning.

Shampooing/ Neutralizing   When the hair is thoroughly rinsed, neutralize it as directed by your instructor. Most manufacturers provide a neutralizing shampoo that is applied to the hair after rinsing. Others prescribe the use of a non-alkaline or cream shampoo, sometimes followed by a neutralizer.

Gently work the shampoo into the hair. Use care to avoid tangling the hair or breaking any fragile ends. Manipulate the shampoo by working with the fingers underneath the hair, not on top. Use warm water to rinse and keep the hair straight. Repeat the shampoo until the hair lathers well and all the relaxer is removed (Figure 7-13).

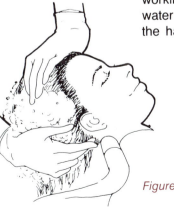

Figure 7.-13. Shampooing the hair

After shampooing, completely saturate the hair with neutralizer if it is required by the manufacturer. Beginning in the nape, carefully comb with a wide-tooth comb, working upward toward the forehead. Use the comb to:

1. Keep the hair straight
2. Ensure complete saturation with the neutralizer
3. Remove any tangles without pulling

Time the neutralizer as directed and rinse thoroughly. Towel blot gently. Condition the hair as necessary, then proceed with styling. Discard used supplies. Cleanse and sanitize equipment; wash and sanitize your hands. Fill out a record card of all timings and treatments during the service and file the card.

Alternate method: Another way to cleanse the hair after rinsing out the relaxer would be with conditioner. Apply the conditioner and massage into the scalp as you would shampoo. Rinse and repeat the procedure to distribute conditioner with a fine-tooth comb. Cover the client's head with a plastic cap and seat him or her under the dryer. This is an advanced technique. Be guided by your instructor and the manufacturer's directions. Rinse and repeat the conditioning.

Conditioners and Conditioner Fillers

Many manufacturers recommend that you apply a conditioner before setting the hair to offset the harshness of the sodium hydroxide in the relaxer and help restore some of the natural oils of the scalp and hair. Many types of conditioners are available.

Cream-type Conditioners. These are applied to the scalp and hair, then carefully rinsed out. The hair is then towel dried. Apply setting lotion; set the hair on rollers; dry and style the hair in the usual manner.

Protein-type (Liquid) Conditioners. These are applied to the scalp and hair prior to setting and allowed to remain in the hair to serve as a setting lotion. Set the hair on rollers, then dry and style in the usual manner.

> *Note:* Because of the fragile condition of the hair, it is advisable to wind the hair on rollers without extreme tension.

Conditioner Fillers. These are often required before the chemical relaxer can be used. The conditioner filler, usually a protein product, is applied to the entire head of hair when dry. It protects overporous or slightly damaged hair from being overprocessed on any part of the hair shaft and permits uniform distribution and action of the chemical relaxer.

To receive complete benefits from the conditioner filler, rub it gently onto the hair from the scalp to the hair ends, using either the hands or a comb (Figure 7-14). Then towel dry the hair or use a cool dryer to completely dry the hair.

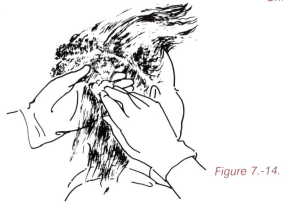

Figure 7.-14.

SODIUM HYDROXIDE RETOUCH

To process the new growth that will eventually appear on the head of a client with relaxed hair, follow all the steps for a regular relaxing treatment with one exception: **The relaxer is applied only to the new growth** (Figure 7-15).

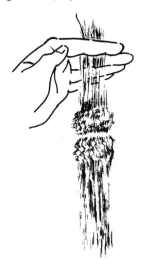

Figure 7-15.

In order to avoid breakage of previously treated hair, apply a cream conditioner over the hair that received the earlier treatment, thus avoiding overlapping damage (Figure 7-16).

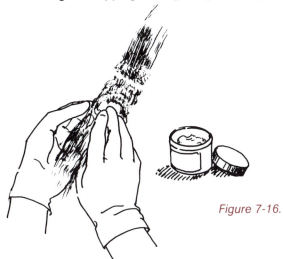

Figure 7-16.

RELAXING PROCESS WITH AMMONIUM THIOGLYCOLATE

Ammonium thioglycolate *(a-MOHN-i-um thi-o-GLI-ko-lay* **(also called thio relaxer)** is the same type of product used in co[l] waving, with a heavy cream or gel added to the formula to kee[p] the hair straight.

As in cold waving, the relaxer breaks the sulfur and hydroge[n] bonds, softening and swelling the hair. By the mechanical actio[n] of the hands, brush, or fingers, the hair is smoothed and held i[n] a straightened position.

When the hair is straightened, the neutralizer is applied to it (servin[g] the same purpose as the neutralizer in cold waving). It re-forms th[e] sulfur and hydrogen bonds and rehardens the hair in its new[l] straightened position.

Manufacturers vary their products according to the texture an[d] condition of the hair. Tinted and lightened hair requires a weake[r] formula.

Thio relaxers have a milder relaxing action on curly hair than sodiu[m] hydroxide relaxers. You may choose them for finely textured ha[ir] or when it is desirable to remove less curl from the hair. Thio relaxer[s] can also be used to reduce excessive curl formed in a permane[nt] wave. Consult your instructor for directions and precautions for th[is] specialized service.

Techniques for thio type relaxers vary. The general procedur[e] involves preparing the hair (gently shampooing if necessary), applyin[g] a base if necessary, applying the relaxer in the manner outline[d] under "Relaxing Process with Sodium Hydroxide," and strand testin[g.] Directions vary greatly at this point, so read the manufacturer['s] instructions carefully. Remove the relaxer from the hair and neutraliz[e] as directed; then condition and proceed with styling. As with an[y] chemical service, exercise great caution so that the hair is n[ot] excessively heated or stretched during styling; this can damage th[e] hair.

Thio Retouch

Hair treated with thio relaxers might require a retouch after regrowt[h] is apparent. If so, follow all steps for a regular thio hair relaxin[g] treatment, with the exception of the relaxer which is applied on[ly] to the new growth (Figure 7-17). Conditioner should be applied t[o] the previously relaxed hair to protect it from damage.

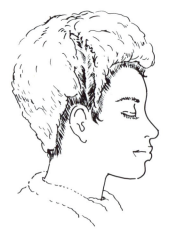

Figure 7-17.

Other Relaxers   Recently, researchers have developed acid relaxers for the treatment of excessively curly hair. Like acid permanent waves, the relaxer works with bisulfites rather than with thioglycolate acid. This type of relaxer is designed as a milder acting one, much like the thio. Some can also be used as a prewrap preparation for performing a soft curl permanent wave on Black hair.

> *Note:* Calcium hydroxide products have become popular in the salon; they are called *no lye* relaxers. This title is misleading because the products do contain lye but in lesser proportions than sodium hydroxide relaxers. Because of the lesser percentage of lye in calcium hydroxide relaxers, they do not completely close the cuticle of the hair and often leave a client's hair frizzy instead of smooth, and make it dry and dull.

SAFETY PRECAUTIONS

1. Examine the scalp for abrasions; if any are present, do not give a hair relaxing treatment.
2. Analyze the hair; give a strand test.
3. Do not shampoo the hair prior to the application of a sodium hydroxide product.
4. Do not apply a sodium hydroxide relaxer over a thio relaxer.
5. Do not apply a thio relaxer over a sodium hydroxide relaxer.
6. Never use a strong relaxer on fine hair; it can cause breakage.
7. Thermal irons may be used on chemically relaxed hair. Do not use excessive heat because it can cause damage relaxed hair.
8. Do not relax damaged hair. Instead, suggest a series of conditioning treatments.
9. Apply a protective base to avoid burning or irritating the scalp with the sodium hydroxide relaxer.
10. Wear protective gloves.
11. Protect the client's eyes.
12. Use extreme care when applying the relaxer to avoid accidentally spreading it on the ears, scalp, or skin.
13. Test the action of the relaxer frequently to determine how fast the natural curl is being removed.
14. Be sure to thoroughly remove the relaxer from the hair. Failure to do so will permit the relaxer to continue to process, resulting in hair damage. Direct a stream of warm water from the scalp to the hair ends.
15. Do not remove your protective gloves until all the relaxer has been removed. When rinsing the shampoo from the hair, always work from the scalp to the ends to prevent tangling.
16. Use a wide-tooth comb and avoid pulling when combing the hair after the relaxation process is complete. Avoid scratching the scalp with the comb or your fingernails.
17. Apply a conditioner to the scalp and hair before setting.
18. When retouching the new growth, do not allow the relaxer to overlap onto the hair already straightened.

19. Do not give a hair relaxing treatment to hair treated with a metallic dye.

20. At the completion of each treatment, fill out a client record card.

21. Have the client sign a release statement to protect the salon and the cosmetologist.

22. It is not advisable to use chemical relaxers on lightened hair.

QUESTIONS FOR REVIEW

1. How do sodium hydroxide and neutralizer chemically affect the hair?

2. What are the three basic relaxing steps?

3. What is the procedure for a relaxer test?

4. What are the steps in the procedure for relaxing with sodium hydroxide?

5. How does a conditioner filler work?

6. What is the procedure for the sodium hydroxide retouch?

7. How does ammonium thioglycolate differ from sodium hydroxide in its effect on curly hair?

8. What is a third type of relaxer?

9. What are 18 safety precautions to be taken in chemical relaxing?

Chapter 8 Soft Curl Permanent Waving

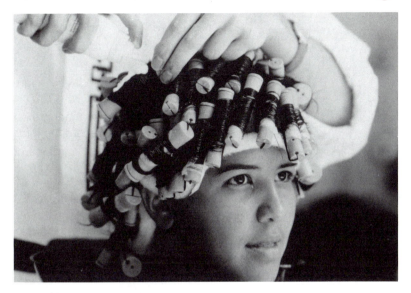

LEARNING OBJECTIVES

After you have mastered this chapter, you will be able to:

1. Give seven safety tips for soft curl permanent waving.
2. List what information you will need on a client record card.
3. Give the procedure for a soft curl permanent wave.
4. Describe the aftercare of soft curl permanently waved hair.

INTRODUCTION

Soft curl permanent waving is a method of permanently waving Black or excessively curly hair. It is known by various names according to the manufacturers of the products being used. The purpose of soft curl permanent waving is to restructure the curl pattern into a looser, more uniform curl size and a direction that is more manageable for styling. Soft curl permanent waving (or restructuring) is different from chemically relaxing hair in that chemical relaxing arranges hair in a straighter pattern and soft curl permanent waving reshapes or elongates the natural curls.

SAFETY TIPS

Before beginning the soft curl permanent waving service, the following safety tips should be considered. Soft curl permanent waves contain ammonium thioglycolate, the chemical present in regular permanent waves and some chemical relaxers.

1. Do not give a soft curl permanent wave to hair that has been relaxed with sodium hydroxide.
2. Do not use a soft curl permanent wave on hair that has been colored with metallic dye or compound henna.
3. Always recondition hair that is bleached, tinted or damaged until it is sufficiently strong to ensure that the soft curl service will not cause further damage.
4. If waving lotion or neutralizer accidentally gets into the client's eyes, flush the eyes immediately with water and refer the client to a physician right away.

5. Always follow the manufacturer's instructions. Otherwise, poor results and damage to the client's hair and skin might result. Consult with your instructor whenever you are unsure of the procedure.

6. Use a protective base cream around the client's hairline, ears, and neck.

7. Take frequent test curls to ensure proper curl formation without damage.

8. Before giving a soft curl permanent wave, thoroughly analyze the hair and scalp and record the information for future services.

9. Complete client record cards carefully and accurately.

CLIENT RECORD CARDS

Complete records for each client will help ensure the best possible service. You'll have to refer to these cards when the client comes back for additional services. The illustration shows an example of the information you will need on a client record card (Figure 8-1).

RELAXER RECORD

Name . . . . Tel. . . . .

Address . . . . City . . . .

DESCRIPTION OF HAIR

Form	Length	Texture		Pororosity	
☐ wavy	☐ short	☐ coarse	☐ soft	☐ very porous	☐ less porous
☐ curly	☐ medium	☐ medium	☐ silky	☐ moderately porous	☐ least porous
☐ extra-curly	☐ long	☐ fine	☐ wiry	☐ normal	☐ resistant

Condition:

☐ virgin   ☐ retouch   ☐ dry   ☐ oily   ☐ lightened

Tinted with . . . .

Previously relaxed with (name of relaxer) . . . .

☐ Original sample of hair enclosed   ☐ not enclosed

TYPE OF SOFT CURL PERMANENT

☐ whole head   ☐ retouch

☐ relaxer . . . .   strength . . . .   ☐ straightener . . . . strength . . . .

Results

☐ good   ☐ poor   ☐ sample of hair enclosed   ☐ not enclosed

Date	Operator	Price	Date	Operator	Price
. . . .			. . . .		
. . . .			. . . .		
. . . .			. . . .		

Figure 8.-1. Record card

SOFT CURL PERMANENT WAVE APPLICATION

Now you are ready to give a soft curl permanent wave. Soft curl perms are versatile in that they can dry naturally for a wet look, be blown dry and curled for a casual look, or be wet set for a more formal look.

Implements and Materials

Record card	Timer
Shampoo cape	Applicators
Neck strips and towels	Curling rods
Mild shampoo	Porous end papers
Combs	Prewrap solution
Gloves	Waving lotion, gel, or cream
Protective base cream	Cotton or neutralizing bands
Neutralizer	Plastic bag or cap
Styling lotion	Plastic hair clips
(curl activator)	Spray bottle
Scissors or razor	Picks
Conditioners	

Preparation

1. Examine the client's scalp. Do not use permanent waving products if the scalp shows signs of cuts, abrasions, or scratches, or if the client has experienced an allergic reaction to a previous curl.

2. Test the hair for porosity and elasticity (see chapter 7, Chemical Hair Relaxing).

3. Shampoo and rinse the hair thoroughly with a mild shampoo. Towel dry, leaving the hair damp.

4. Apply a liquid protein conditioner to the hair, leave on for 10 minutes, then rinse well. (Manufacturer's directions might omit this step or differ from this step. Be guided by your instructor.)

5. Remove tangles with a large-tooth comb (Figure 8-2).

6. Part the hair into four or five sections, as recommended by your instructor. Hold sections in place with plastic clips (Figure 8-3).

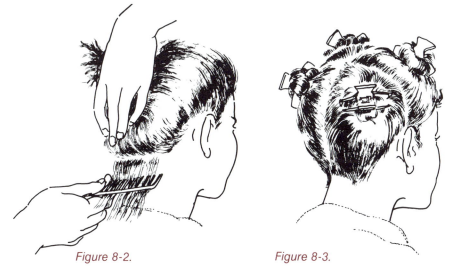

Figure 8-2.   *Figure 8-3.*

Note: If the manufacturer recommends it, put a protective cream on the entire scalp, including around the hairline.

Procedure
1. Put on protective gloves.
2. Apply thio gel or cream to one section at a time, using the back of a comb, hair coloring brush, or the fingers (Figure 8-4). Use the tail of the comb or brush to part the hair and begin the application of thio gel or cream to the hair nearest the scalp, starting at the nape or most resistant area. Avoid directly contacting the scalp with the thio to prevent irritation. Work the thio gel or cream through to the ends of the hair.
3. Comb the thio product through the entire head, first with a wide-tooth comb, then with a smaller-tooth comb (Figure 8-5).

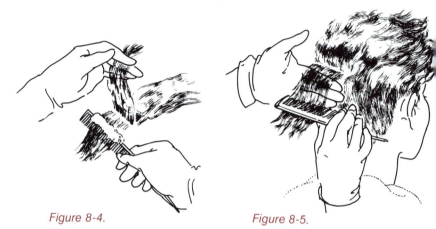

Figure 8-4.   Figure 8-5.

4. When the hair becomes supple and flexible (Figure 8-6), rinse with lukewarm water and towel dry. Take extra care not to tangle the hair. Some manufacturers do not recommend removal of the thio product by rinsing. Read the instructions and check with your instructor.
5. Section the hair into nine sections (Figure 8-7) as directed by your instructor. Subsection as you wrap the hair.
6. Wrap the hair as desired on curling rods, using two papers for each curl. For fragile hair, continue using as many papers as necessary to protect the hair all the way to the scalp. This is done to prevent the bands of the rods from breaking the hair. (Your instructor's directions might vary.)

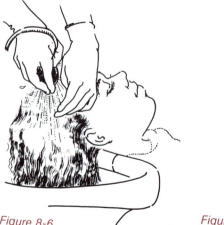

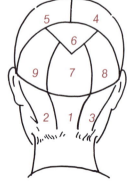

Figure 8-6.   Figure 8-7.

7. In order to rearrange the curl pattern of the hair, select a rod at least two times larger than the natural curl. To achieve a good curl formation, the hair should encircle the rod at least 2 1/2 times (Figure 8-8).

8. After the wrap has been completed, protect the client's skin by placing cotton around the hairline and neck (Figure 8-9). Reapply protective base cream around the hairline.

9. Apply the thio gel, cream, or lotion to all the curls until they are thoroughly saturated (Figure 8-10). Remove the saturated cotton. (Alternative method: If the manufacturer's directions have not called for the thio product to be rinsed out at this point, spray each curl with liquid waving lotion to reactivate the thio product.)

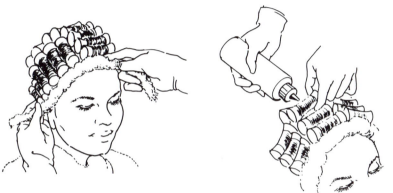

Figure 8-8.

Figure 8-9.

Figure 8-10.

10. Cover the client's head with a plastic cap or bag.

11. Have the client sit under a preheated dryer for 15 to 25 minutes (set timer) or as recommended by the manufacturer (Figure 8-11).

12. Take a test curl (Figure 8-12) by unwinding the rod 1 1/2 times without pulling on the hair. Rewind the test curl and continue to check the curl pattern at regular intervals.

13. When the desired curl pattern has been reached, spray the hair with liquid protein conditioner and place the client under the dryer for 10 minutes more. Manufacturer's instructions might vary on when to apply the conditioner. Check with your instructor.

14. Rinse the hair thoroughly with warm water (Figure 8-13). Blot each curl with a towel to absorb excess moisture.

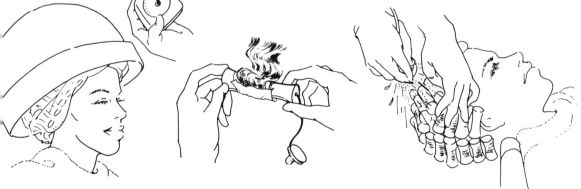

Figure 8-11.

Figure 8-12.

Figure 8-13.

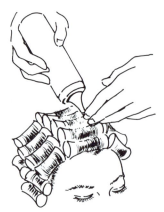

Figure 8-14.

15. Use a prepared neutralizer or mix neutralizer as directed by the manufacturer. Saturate each curl twice (Figure 8-14). Allow the neutralizer to remain on the curls for 5 to 10 minutes or as directed by the manufacturer.

16. Carefully remove the rods and apply the balance of the neutralizer to the hair. Work the neutralizer through with the fingers for thorough distribution (Figure 8-15) and allow it to remain on the hair as directed. Some manufacturers recommend a thorough rinsing while the hair is still wrapped on rods. Check with your instructor.

17. Rinse the hair thoroughly with cool water and towel dry.

18. Trim and shape the hair to the desired style (Figure 8-16).

19. Apply conditioner (if you did not do so in step 12).

20. Air dry hair or style as directed (Figures 8-17 and 8-18).

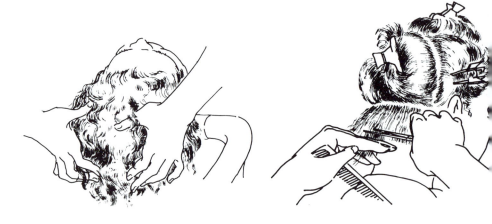

Figure 8-15.   *Figure 8-16.*

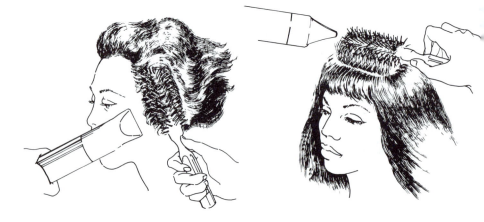

Figure 8-17.   *Figure 8-18.*

Alternate Soft Curl Procedure--The Body Wrap

1. Apply a pre-wrap solution or conditioner to hair.
2. Using the tail of a comb, section the hair, clipping each section up so it does not interfere with the wrap.
3. Divide the sections into subsections that are no larger than the length and diameter of the rod selected.
4. Begin wrapping the hair on rods in an off-base position, with one end paper on top of the subsection and one below (Figure 8-19), starting at the back of the head.

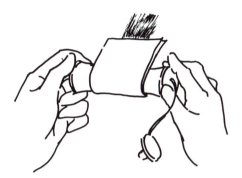

Figure 8-19.

5. Slide the end papers to the end of the subsection.
6. Wind the rod evenly to the scalp so that the hair is smooth, resembling thread on a spool.
7. Move from the back of the head and begin winding the rods from the front of the head back to the crown.
8. Place the rods at the right side and then the left side of the head.
9. Apply protective cream around the client's hairline and attach protective cotton (Figure 8-20).

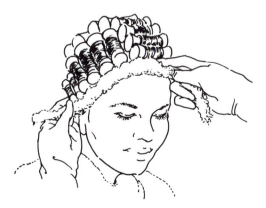

Figure 8-20.

10. Put on your protective gloves.
11. Pour the proper strength perm wave lotion into applicator bottle
12. Start applying lotion to the most resistant area, usually the nape
13. Saturate each rod and gently press into it with your finger (Figure 8-21).

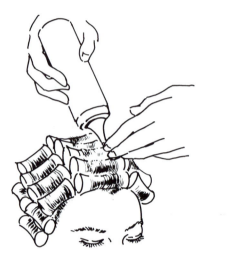

Figure 8-21.

14. Remove the saturated cotton from the hairline.
15. Blot lotion from one curl to test for the desired S-shaped pattern

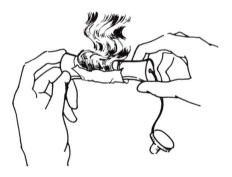

Figure 8-22.

16. Unroll the curl several turns to test it (Figure 8-22).
17. Reroll the curl and check frequently at different places on the head, for desired curl. When the hair is very porous, you might have to check the test curls as often as every 30 seconds.
18. If hair is particularly resistant, showing little change after 15 minutes of processing, apply a second application of lotion and continue to process.

19. Rinse or blot the lotion from the rods according to the manufacturer's or your instructor's directions. (Figure 8-23).
20. If the product calls for removing the lotion with water, make sure the water is tepid.
21. Blot away excess water to ensure proper absorption of the neutralizer.
22. Apply the neutralizer in the same manner that the lotion was applied (Figure 8-24).

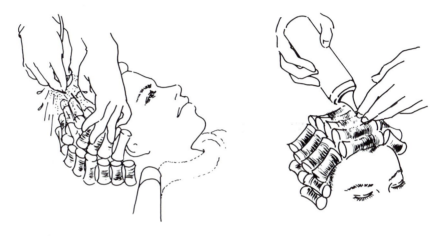

Figure 8-23.   *Figure 8-24.*

23. Carefully time the neutralization.
24. When neutralization is complete, rinse the hair thoroughly with cool water (Figure 8-25).

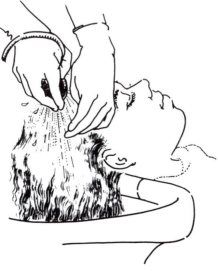

Figure 8-25.

25. Gently remove the rods without stretching the newly formed curls (Figure 8-26).
26. Close the cuticle with a finishing rinse.
27. Rinse with water and towel dry.
28. Style the hair, avoiding excess heat or stretching.

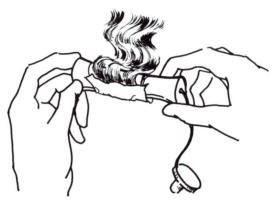

Figure 8-26.

AFTERCARE OF SOFT CURL PERMANENT WAVED HAIR

To ensure that the soft curl permanent wave remains looking healthy and pretty, the following steps should be taken:

1. For a natural look, never comb or brush the curls when wet. Use a lifting pick instead.
2. Shampoo as often as necessary, using a mild shampoo.
3. Conditioner or curl activator should be used daily to maintain flexibility, sheen, and proper moisture balance of the hair.

QUESTIONS FOR REVIEW

1. What are seven safety tips for soft curl permanent waving?
2. What information will you need on a client record card?
3. What is the procedure for a soft curl permanent wave?
4. What are the three steps of aftercare for a soft curl permanent wave?

Chapter 9 Thermal Styling

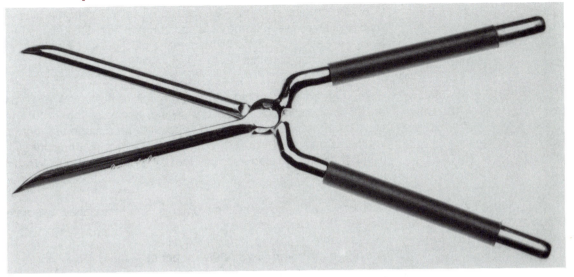

LEARNING OBJECTIVES   After you have mastered this chapter, you will be able to:

1. Give the procedures for both straightening and curling with blow-dry styling.
2. List four safety precautions for blow-dry styling.
3. Give the procedures for both thermal waving and thermal curling chemically relaxed hair.
4. List the five types of curls that can be achieved with the curling iron.
5. Give ten hints and reminders for thermal waving and curling
6. Give the procedure for pressing.
7. List five safety precautions for pressing.

INTRODUCTION   To be successful, the cosmetologist must master the art of thermal styling and understand its theory. Blow-dryers and curling irons are used to produce both curly and straight styles on Black hair. A pressing comb is used to straighten hair.

BLOW-DRY STYLING   Blow-dry styling is basically the technique of drying and styling damp hair in one operation. This technique creates the basic structure of hairstyles without time-consuming setting, drying, and combing.

The Blow-Dryer   The blow-dryer is an electrical device especially designed for drying and styling hair in a single operation. Its main parts are a handle, nozzle, small fan, heating element, and controls (Figure 9-1).

When in operation, the blow-dryer produces a steady stream of temperature-controlled air. The controls permit the stylist to make necessary heat adjustments while operating the dryer. The wattage on a blow-dryer for use on Black hair should be between 1,200 and 1,500.

Caution: Make sure the blow-dryer is perfectly clean and free of dirt, grease, and hair before using. Debris within the blow-dryer can cause extreme heat and burn the hair. If the air intake at the back side of the blow-dryer is blocked, the element in the dryer can burn out.

Straightening and Curling with the Blow-Dryer

You can both straighten and curl the hair using a blow-dryer and brush or comb. Before blow-dry styling, check to make sure the client's hair is in good condition. If not, it is recommended that you set the client's hair with rollers and style. Continue conditioning the client's hair during salon visits until the hair is in good enough condition for blow-dry styling.

Equipment, Implements, and Materials Needed for Blow-Dry Styling

The following equipment, implements, and materials are required for blow-dry styling:

- Blow-dryer (1,200 to 1,500 wattage)
- Wide-tooth comb (hard rubber or bone)
- Styling agent
- Conditioner
- Hair spray or fixative
- Vent brush

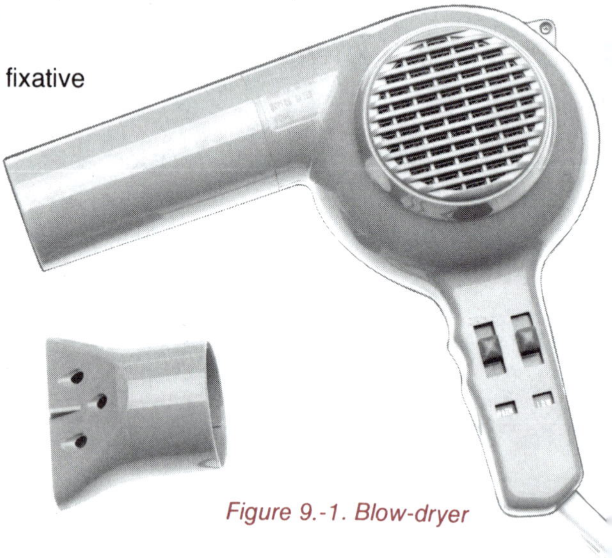

Figure 9.-1. Blow-dryer

Note: Never use a plastic comb in blow-dry styling because it can melt under the heat of the dryer.

Procedure for Straightening with Blow-Dry Styling

1. Divide the hair into four sections (nose to nape and ear to ear) using a wide-tooth comb or vent brush (Figure 9-2).
2. Beginning at the nape area, insert the comb into a thin subsection of hair, turning the comb slightly to place tension on the hair (Figure 9-3).
3. Begin to move the comb slowly down the subsection of hair, following closely with the blow-dryer on high heat, 3 or 4 inches away from the hair (Figure 9-4). The dryer should always follow the comb, working in the direction of the desired style. Always start at the foundation of the style so you are blowing damp hair onto dry hair.

4. Repeat this procedure as many times as necessary to dry the hair and to achieve the desired finish.

5. Continue through the four sections, drying both the top and bottom of each subsection. Slight tension must be used for the hair to be dried in its new, straighter form (Figure 9-5).

> **Note:** Since the hair at the hairline is more delicate, handle it carefully to avoid damage.

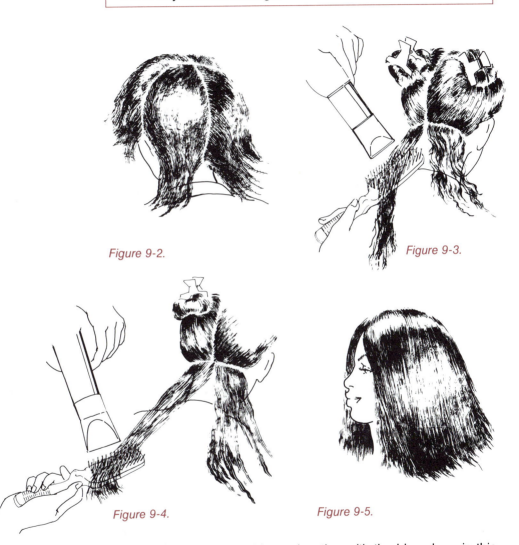

Figure 9-2.

Figure 9-3.

Figure 9-4.

Figure 9-5.

Procedure for Curling with Blow-Dry Styling

A round brush is used in conjunction with the blow-dryer in this procedure (the diameter of the brush used will depend on the amount of curl and direction desired).

1. Properly shape the hair.

2. Apply a styling agent and/or conditioner.

3. Wrap a brush with lamb's wool to prevent tangling. (Some professionals think this step is optional. Be guided by your instructor.)

4. Starting at the crown or top of the head, remove moisture and dry the base of the hair with the blow-dryer, using your fingers to lift the hair from the scalp.

5. Pick up a subsection of hair with the brush (Figure 9-6).

6. Brush the hair away from the face, following the direction of the brush with the blower, until the hair slides easily through the brush (Figure 9-7). Remember to keep the brush in constant motion while heat is on the hair and to follow the brush with the dryer. (This will prevent the hair from burning and give it shine and gloss.)

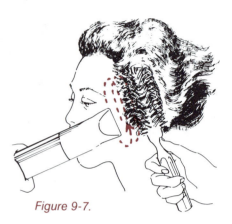

Figure 9-6.

Figure 9-7.

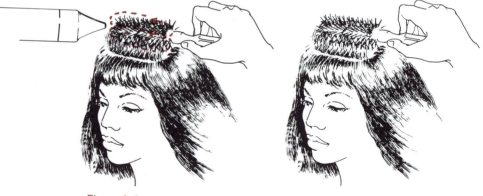

Figure 9-8.

Figure 9-9.

7. As a subsection dries, roll the hair around the brush to the scalp (Figure 9-8). Finish drying with the blower, using a slow back-and-forth motion (Figure 9-9).

8. Let the hair cool completely before removing the brush.

9. Clip, curl or secure it with a roller if desired.

Note: This procedure is not very successful on hair that has been completely relaxed. Relaxed hair is more successfully curled with an electric curling iron.

Other Effects Achieved with Blow-Dry Styling

There are three other effects you can create on Black hair using the blow-dryer.

Minimum volume. This effect is used in flatter or close-to-the-head styles. Begin drying at the root area and proceed to the ends, remembering to keep the brush or comb and blow-dryer in continuous motion while heat is directed on the hair. Always keep the brush or comb at the top of the head to create movability.

Fullness with minimum bend. Dry the hair in the opposite direction of its finished style with the brush or comb and blow-dryer kept underneath a subsection to create volume. Return hair to its styled position and complete to give texture and fullness.

Texture and fullness. The amount of texture and fullness in a style can be created and controlled by applying tension to subsections of the hair with the hands, brush, or comb.

SAFETY PRECAUTIONS FOR BLOW-DRYING

To ensure both your safety and that of the client and his or her hair, the following precautions should be observed:

1. Follow the brush or comb with the blow-dryer, working in the direction of the desired style and blowing damp hair onto dry hair.
2. Blow hair away from the scalp to prevent burns.
3. Test the temperature controls.
4. Check the brush bristles for sharp points.
5. Apply a protective setting agent to the hair to shield it from the heat of the blow-dryer.
6. Place the client under a warm dryer or blow dry the hair to remove excess moisture. This will minimize the damage of stretching chemically treated hair.

STYLING CHEMICALLY RELAXED HAIR WITH A CURLING IRON

A popular way to give style and fullness to chemically relaxed hair is with an electric (Figure 9-10) or stove-heated curling iron (Figure 9-11).

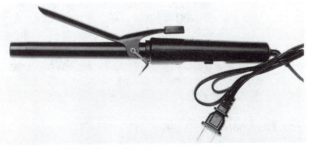

Figure 9-10. Electric curling iron.

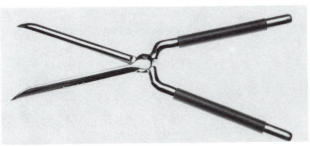

Figure 9-11. Stove-heated curling iron.

Using the Curling Iron

The temperature of the curling iron will depend on the texture and condition of the Black client's hair. Coarse hair, as a rule, can stand more heat than fine hair. Test the temperature of the curling iron by clamping it over a piece of tissue paper and holding for 5 seconds. If the paper scorches or turns brown, the iron is too hot.

Preparation

Take the iron in hand, using the third and middle fingers to control the scissor-like clicking action that releases the hair. Use the index and middle fingers to control the turning of the iron (Figure 9-12). The thumb rests on the stem of the iron to provide support and balance while the iron is manipulated on the hair subsection. Proper holding, turning, and clicking of the iron should be practiced regularly until it becomes natural. Use a cold iron to practice.

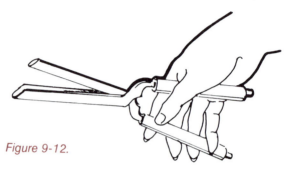

Figure 9-12.

Note: Keep the styling comb in hand at all times when working with the curling iron so that it will not be clamped flat on the subsection, creating a ridge or buckle.

After the hair has been thoroughly shampooed, conditioned, and towel dried, take the client to the styling chair and apply a blow-drying solution. Comb the solution through the hair to distribute evenly. Comb the hair in the direction of the planned style. Place the client under a warm dryer to remove moisture. After 50 percent of the moisture has been removed, use the blow-dryer to remove the remaining moisture and establish a style foundation. Now you are ready to use the curling iron.

Procedure For Thermal Waving Chemically Relaxed Hair

1. With a comb, pick up a 2 inch wide subsection of hair.
2. Take the subsection between the index and middle fingers, making sure the hair is spread evenly (Figure 9-13).
3. Insert the iron with the rod on top (Figure 9-14).
4. Close the iron and insert the comb into a subsection, slightly below the iron.
5. Draw the iron 1/4 inch to the right and draw the comb 1/4 inch to the left (Figure 9-15).
6. Holding the comb and iron in this position, roll up the iron one quarter of a turn (Figure 9-16).
7. Let the hair heat.

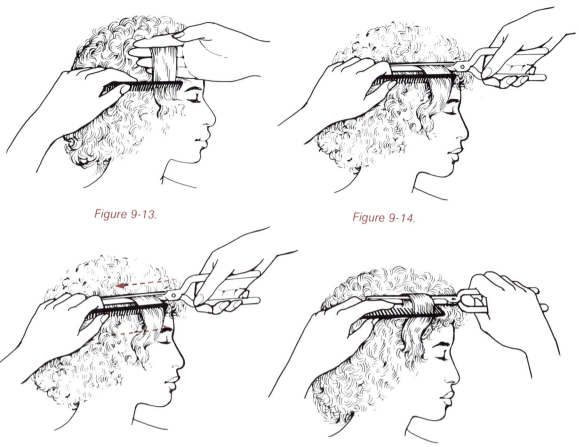

Figure 9-13.

Figure 9-14.

Figure 9-15.

Figure 9-16.

8. Open the iron and slide it down the subsection of hair until the groove of the iron is directly underneath the wave just completed (Figure 9-17).

9. Draw the iron 1/4 inch to the right and the comb 1/4 inch to the left (Figure 9-18).

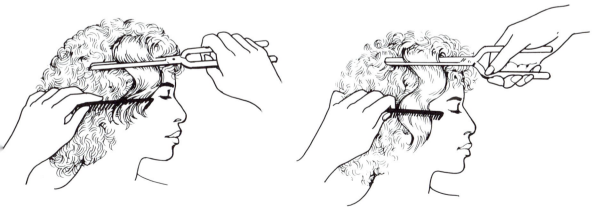

Figure 9-17.

Figure 9-18.

10. Roll up the iron one quarter of a turn (Figure 9-19).
11. Let the hair heat.
12. Slide the iron down the subsection until the top of its groove is directly underneath the wave just completed (Figure 9-20).
13. Repeat all steps in the procedure until the entire subsection is waved.

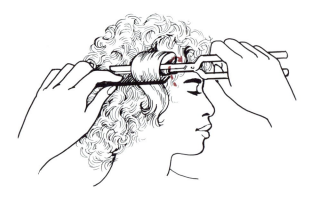

Figure 9-19.

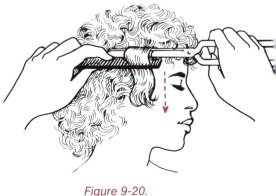

Figure 9-20.

Procedure for Thermal Curling Chemically Relaxed Hair

1. Divide the hair into five sections. The first section, about 2-1/2 inches wide, extends from the center of the forehead to the nape. Divide two side panels in half, from the top parting to neck, to provide four additional sections.
2. Subdivide the sections into subsections—each approximately 3/4 inches to 2-1/2 inches wide.
3. Begin the curl formation by inserting the iron into a hair subsection about 1/2 inch away from the scalp (Figure 9-21). Use slight tension to wrap the subsection over the iron.
4. Hold in this position for a few seconds to establish a base. Keep the iron slightly open to prevent crimping the hair (Figure 9-22). To avoid *fish hooks* be sure to control the ends at all times. The subsection should lie flat, and the ends should be fed completely into the iron (Figure 9-23).

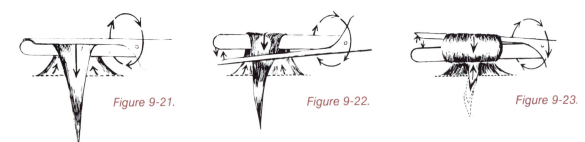

Figure 9-21.   Figure 9-22.   Figure 9-23.

5. After forming a strong, smooth curl movement at the base, slide up the subsection until you can rotate the iron one full turn.
6. Make one complete turn of the iron so that it is resting on the base of the curl with the ends of the subsection kept flat against the iron.

7. Continue in this manner until the ends are fed inside the iron. Make sure the ends of the subsections lie flat on the iron to insure a smooth, even curl. This is extremely important to remember. When turning the iron, keep the hair within the width of the subsection.

8. Hold the hair in the iron for approximately 10 seconds.

9. Carefully withdraw the iron from the curl, using a clicking, scissor-like movement to release the hair.

10. Secure the curl in place with a clip or velcro roller.

Using the Curling Iron on Short and Medium-Length Hair

The base of the curl is formed in the usual manner, taking a thin subsection of hair held at the desired angle and holding the iron at the base for approximately 5 seconds. Hold the subsection toward you with a minimum degree of tension. After 5 seconds, begin to rotate the iron in a clockwise motion. Open and close the iron rapidly to avoid permanent creases created in the hair by the clamp of the iron. Continue to rotate the irons in a clockwise position as you guide the ends of the subsection into the center of the curl.

CURL TYPES

There are five types of curls you can create with the curling iron: volume-base curls, full-base curls, half-base curls, off-base curls, and thermal flat curls.

Volume-Base Curls

Volume-base curls provide maximum lift or volume, because the curl is placed very high on the base (Figure 9-24).

Hold the section of hair 135 degrees forward from the top of the base parting and place the curling iron in the subsection, 1/2 inch from the scalp with a slight degree of tension. Wrap the subsection over the shaft of the iron and hold it in this position for about 5 seconds. You will notice a strong base formation through the use of this technique. After the strong base is formed, continue to rotate the iron to complete the curl, making sure the ends of the subsection are fed directly into the center of the curl.

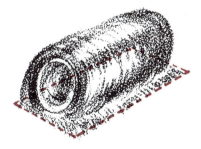

Figure 9-24. Volume-base curl.

Full-Base Curls

Full-base curls provide a strong curl with full volume.

The same procedure is followed as for the volume-base curl, except that the hair is held 125 degrees above the top of the base parting. You then proceed in the same manner as with the volume-base curl.

Half-Base Curls

Half-base curls provide curls with moderate lift or volume. They are used to blend between style lines (Figure 9-25).

Proceed again with the same method as above, except hold the subsection at a 90-degree angle or straight out from the head. Always make sure that the hair is fed directly into the center of the curl.

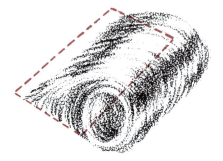

Figure 9-25. Full-base curl.

Off-Base Curls

Off-base curls provide curls with only slight lift or volume. They give maximum mobility (Figure 9-26).

Proceed as in the method above, but hold the hair 70 degrees up from the head. The half- and off-base curls do not have as strong a base as the volume- or full-base curls. Insert the iron for a few seconds before completing the curl.

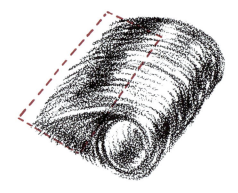

Figure 9-26. Off-base curl.

Thermal Flat Curls

This advanced technique creates pin curls with thermal equipment. For this curl, the base is first established by inserting the iron about 1/4 inch from the scalp. Use care to avoid burning the client with the iron. Hold the base of the curl with the index finger as the iron is swiveled around in the direction of the curl. Be sure that the ends of the subsection are in the center of the curl, around the iron. Next, insert the large teeth of the comb into the subsection at the base of the curl. This will hold the base and protect the client. Carefully open and close the clamp of the iron until the curl is completed. Remove the iron and reposition the curl either into an on-base or off-base flat pin curl. Clip the curl at the base and allow it to cool.

REMINDERS AND HINTS FOR THERMAL WAVING AND CURLING

The following hints and reminders are especially important for the cosmetologist to keep in mind when working with Black hair.

1. Always test your curling iron on a neck strip before starting your style. Grasp the strip with the heated iron and hold for a few seconds. If the iron burns or scorches the paper, it is too hot.

2. For stove-heated irons, be sure to recheck the temperature of the iron before forming each curl.

3. The comb serves as an insulator to protect the client from burns. Always use the comb in this manner when curling around the ears and face.

4. When curling short hair, rest the iron on the comb to produce a curl that is tight and close to the scalp.

5. Constantly practice these important actions with thermal irons: Opening and closing the iron in a quick clicking action to release the hair and eliminate binding, and turning the iron.

6. Develop a smooth, even rotating action while opening and closing the iron at regular intervals.

7. Dry hair before applying heat with the thermal iron.

8. Keep in mind that less heat and less time might be required for thermal curling fine, bleached, tinted, permed, or relaxed hair. Your instructor will help you test the condition of a client's hair to see if thermal iron styling is the best method.

9. Always keep the subsection smooth on the iron; never twist the ends.

10. Remember to work with small sections and repeat the curling action rather than leave the iron in contact with the hair for more than a few seconds.

11. Turn the subsection and the iron simultaneously to create a perfect curl.

12. Choose the thickness of a subsection according to the texture and condition of the hair and the amount of curl desired.

13. Always allow the hair to cool completely before attempting to style hair. Hot hair that is combed out will lose up to 50 percent of its curl strength.

HAIR PRESSING

Hair pressing is a method of temporarily straightening the hair, using a pressing comb.

Pressing Combs

There are two types of pressing combs: regular and electric (Figure 9-27). They are both constructed of either good quality steel or brass. The handle is usually made of wood, which does not readily absorb heat. The space between the teeth of the comb varies with the size and style of comb. Some combs have more space between the teeth than others. Pressing combs vary in size.

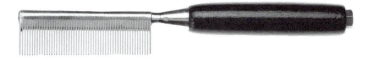

Figure 9-27. Regular pressing comb.

Heating the Pressing Comb

Pressing combs can be heated in gas stoves or electric heaters (Figure 9-28). Electric pressing combs are also available that need only to be plugged into an electrical socket. One type of electric heating comb comes with an on/off switch. Another has a thermostat with a control switch that indicates high or low degrees of heat.

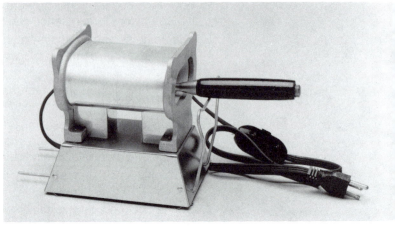

Figure 9-28. Electric heater

Pressing Oil or Cream

The application of pressing oil or cream prior to a hair pressing treatment helps prepare the hair for pressing. Both products have the following beneficial effects:

- Soften the hair
- Prepare and condition the hair for pressing
- Prevent the hair from burning or scorching
- Prevent hair breakage
- Condition the hair after pressing
- Add sheen to pressed hair

Equipment, Implements, and Materials Needed For Pressing

The following equipment, implements, and materials are required for hair pressing:

Pressing comb
Heating appliance (if either a stove- or electrically-heated type of comb are used)
Pressing oil or cream
Brush and comb
Shampoo
Towels and cape
Spatula
Neck strips
Thermal iron

Preparation

To prepare the client for hair pressing, thoroughly shampoo and condition the hair, then towel dry. Apply a light pressing cream in the palms of the hands and rub them together. Then work your hands through the client's hair. Part the hair into four sections and comb through from scalp to ends. Clip each section out of the way and begin drying the first section in the nape with a wide-tooth comb and your blow-dryer. It is important to have a dryer with a metal nozzle for this procedure because more heat is generated. The heat acts as a pressing agent and begins the straightening process. Start in the nape area, blowing the hair up and away from the head. When the hair is 90 percent dry, begin the pressing procedure.

Procedure For Pressing

1. Divide the hair into four main sections. Clip each section.
2. Unclip one hair section at a time and divide into smaller sub-sections. Begin working at the crown of the head.
3. If necessary, apply pressing oil or cream evenly and sparingly over the small subsections.
4. Test the temperature of the heated pressing comb on a neck strip.
5. Grasp the subsection with the index finger and thumb, lifting away from the scalp, pulling the hair with slight tension.
6. Insert the pressing comb into the top side of the subsection, as close to the scalp as possible without burning it. Use a continuous motion to avoid burns.
7. Rotate the comb upward quickly so that the subsection wraps itself partly around the comb. The back rod does the pressing.
8. Move the pressing comb slowly toward the ends of the hair, holding the ends as the pressing comb moves through the subsection.
9. Repeat steps 7 and 8 until the subsection has been sufficiently pressed on the top side.
10. Reverse the comb to the bottom of the subsection, pressing once.
11. Move the completed subsection out of the way.
12. If using a stove-heated comb, return it to the stove for a few seconds to reheat for the next subsection. Test the comb on the neck strip, and repeat steps 1 through 12 until the entire back crown has been completed.
13. Move to the side sections and repeat steps 3 through 12.
14. After completing the pressing procedure, press out the fine hair around the hairline, behind the ears, and in the nape.

Caution: Great care must be taken to protect the client's face, neck, ears, and scalp during pressing.

Note: When regular pressing results are not satisfactory, a hard press is recommended. A hard press means the entire pressing procedure is repeated twice on each subsection of the client's head. Great care must be taken when giving a hard press because it can be extremely damaging to the hair.

PRESSING SAFETY PRECAUTIONS

It is very important that the following precautions be taken to insure the safety of both client and cosmetologist during the pressing procedure.

1. Avoid excessive heat or pressure on the hair and scalp. Burn hair, scalp, and skin can be the result of excess heat, overpressing or poor judgment on the part of the cosmetologist.
2. Keep the pressing comb clean and free from carbon at all times.
3. Adjust the temperature of the pressing comb to the texture and condition of the client's hair.
4. Prevent the smoking and burning of hair during pressing by drying the hair completely after shampooing and avoiding excess application of pressing oil over the hair.
5. Use a moderately warm comb to press short hair on the temples and back of the neck.
6. Keep the pressing comb in constant motion while it is inserted in the hair.

QUESTIONS FOR REVIEW

1. What is the procedure for straightening with blow-dry styling? For curling with blow-dry styling?
2. What are four safety precautions for blow-dry styling?
3. What is the procedure for thermal waving chemically relaxed hair? For thermal curling chemically relaxed hair?
4. What are the five types of curls that can be achieved with the curling iron?
5. What are ten hints and reminders for thermal waving and curling?
6. What is the procedure for pressing?
7. What are five safety precautions for pressing?

Chapter 10 Black Skin and its Care

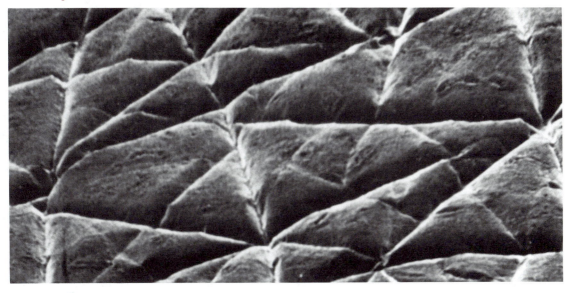

After you have mastered this chapter, you will be able to:

1. Describe the basic structure of the skin.
2. Describe three special characteristics of Black skin.
3. Give the procedure for a facial for oily skin.
4. Describe three skin conditions that affect Black skin.

INTRODUCTION

It is important for the cosmetologist to know the basic structure of the skin and its properties to correctly suggest and administer aesthetic treatments to the client. Being proficient in the practice of professional skin care is yet another way to make clients look and feel better. As interest in skin care grows, so too will client demand for good, professional aesthetic treatment.

THE SKIN

The skin is the largest as well as one of the most important organs of the body (Figure 10-1). A healthy skin is slightly moist, soft and flexible, possesses a slightly acidic reaction, and is free from any disease or disorder. Ideally its texture (feel and appearance) is smooth and fine grained. A fine texture and healthy color indicate a good complexion.

The skin varies in thickness; it is thinnest on the eyelids and thickest on the palms and soles. Continued pressure over any part of the skin can cause it to thicken and develop into a callus.

The skin of the scalp is constructed similarly to the skin elsewhere on the human body. However, the scalp has larger and deeper hair follicles to accommodate the longer hair of the head. (For more information on the scalp and its care see chapter 3, Conditioning.)

Histology of the Skin

The skin contains two main divisions: epidermis and dermis (Figure 10-2). The epidermis is the outermost layer of the skin; the dermis is the underlying or inner layer.

Structures in the Skin

*Figure 10.-1. One Square Inch
of Skin Contains*

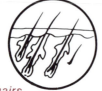

65 hairs

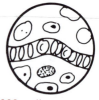

9,500,000 cells

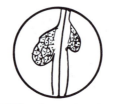

95-100 sebaceous glands

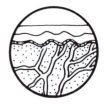

*19 yards (17 meters) of blood
vessels*

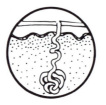

650 sweat glands

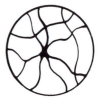

78 yards (70 meters) of nerves

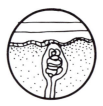

78 sensory apparatuses for heat

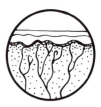

*19,500 sensory cells at the ends
of nerve fibers*

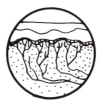

*1,3000 nerve endings to record
pain*

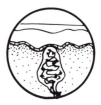

*160-165 pressure apparatuses for
the perception of tactile stimuli*

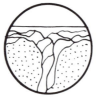

13 sensory apparatuses for cold

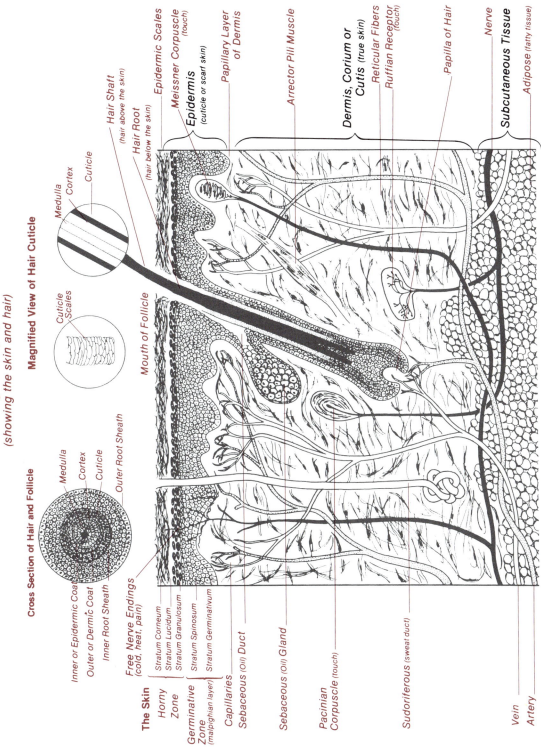

The Integumentary System
(showing the skin and hair)

Cross Section of Hair and Follicle

Magnified View of Hair Cuticle

Medulla
Cortex
Cuticle
Outer Root Sheath
Inner or Epidermic Coat
Outer or Dermic Coat
Inner Root Sheath

Medulla
Cortex
Cuticle

Cuticle
Scales

Free Nerve Endings
(cold, heat, pain)

The Skin

**Horny
Zone**
Stratum Corneum
Stratum Lucidum
Stratum Granulosum

**Germinative
Zone**
(malpighian layer)
Stratum Spinosum
Stratum Germinativum

Capillaries
Sebaceous (oil) Duct
Sebaceous (oil) Gland
Pacinian
Corpuscle *(touch)*
Sudoriferous *(sweat duct)*
Vein
Artery

Mouth of Follicle
Hair Shaft
(hair above the skin)
Hair Root
(hair below the skin)

Epidermic Scales
Meissner Corpuscle
(touch)
Epidermis
(cuticle or scarf skin)
Papillary Layer
of Dermis
Arrector Pili Muscle
**Dermis, Corium or
Cutis** *(true skin)*
Reticular Fibers
Ruffian Receptor
(touch)
Papilla of Hair
Nerve
Subcutaneous Tissue
Adipose *(fatty tissue)*

Figure 10-2.

The **epidermis** *(ep-i-DUR-mis)* is the outer layer of the skin that forms a protective covering over the body. It contains no blood vessels but has many small nerve endings. The epidermis contains the following layers: the **stratum corneum** *(strat-UM kor-nee-um)*, the outer layer of the skin, made up of overlapping cells covered by a thin layer of oil, which helps make this layer almost waterproof; the **stratum lucidum** *(loo-seed-UM)*, which consists of small transparent cells through which light can pass; the **stratum granulosum** *(gran-u-LOH-som)*, which consists of almost dead cells that look like granules and change into a hardened substance; and the **stratum germinativum** *(JUR-mi-na-tiv-um)*, which is composed of several layers of differently shaped cells. The deepest layer contains a dark skin pigment called **melanin** *(mel-a-NIN)*, which protects the sensitive cells below from the destructive effects of sun or artificial light.

The **dermis** *(DUR-mis)* is a highly sensitive and vascular layer of connective tissue. Within the dermis are numerous blood vessels, lymph vessels, nerves, sweat glands, oil glands, hair follicles, arrector pili muscles, and papillae. The dermis consists of the **papillary** *(PAP-i-ler-ee)* layer and the **reticular** *(re-TIK-u-ler)* layer. The papillary layer contains papillae (small, cone-shaped projections of elastic tissue that point upward) and either looped capillaries or nerve fiber endings called tactile corpuscles. This layer also contains melanin. The reticular layer contains: fat cells, blood vessels, lymph vessels, oil glands, sweat glands, hair follicles, and arrector pili muscles.

Subcutaneous *(sub-kyoo-TAY-ni-us)* tissue is a fatty layer found below the dermis. It gives smoothness and contour to the body and contains fats used for both energy and as a protective cushion for the outer skin. Blood and lymph circulate within the subcutaneous tissue to supply nourishment to the skin.

Nerves supplying the skin register basic types of sensations, namely: touch, pain, heat, cold, pressure, or deep touch. Nerve endings are most abundant in the fingertips.

SPECIAL PROPERTIES OF BLACK SKIN

When we understand the unique qualities of individuals, we can better understand the characteristics of Black skin before determining the kinds of skin care treatments that will be best for the client.

Color

Melanin is responsible for the color of the skin. It is dark pigment in the epidermis and hair. **Melanocytes** *(mel-LAN-o-sits)* are melanin-producing cells. Melanocytes in Black skin are more evenly distributed than in Caucasian skin and are larger and more active. The more dense pigmentation in Black skin is an added protection against the damaging effects of the ultraviolet rays of the sun.

Elasticity and Sebaceous Glands

There is a greater elasticity and strength of fibers in the network within the dermis of Black skin. In addition, Black skin usually has more and larger sebaceous glands. These glands provide a built-in moisturizing effect that helps to protect against lines and wrinkles. The aging process is slower and a youthful appearance is often enjoyed well into the mature years of people of color.

Other Special Differences

- Black skin flakes, sheds, and casts off more easily than Caucasian skin.
- Skin cancer is seen less frequently in Black skin due to its deeper pigmentation, which tends to filter out damaging sun radiation.
- Acne is rarely severe in Black people even though there are more sebaceous glands in dark skin.
- The dead cell layer of the epidermis is thicker on Black skin than on Caucasian skin.
- Allergic reactions to products are less frequent in people of color. This is believed to be true because Black skin has a heavier surface cell layer than Caucasian skin.
- Warts are rarely found on Black skin.

Skin Types

There are three major types of skin: oily, dry, and combination. Oily skin looks very shiny and feels slick. Pores are generally enlarged. This type of skin may be susceptible to blackheads, blemishes, and acne.

Dry skin has no shine. It may have a dull and ashen look. The pores are not visible, flakes and dry patches are obvious, and it is easily irritated. Dry skin is prone to lines and wrinkles and is susceptible to premature aging. Obviously dry skin is lacking in moisture or sebum or both.

Combination skin (skin with both dry and oily areas) is quite prevalent among Black people. Combination skin usually has an oily *T* zone with dry areas outside the zone (Figure 10-3). The aim when caring for this type of skin is to normalize both areas through the use of appropriate products and facial treatments.

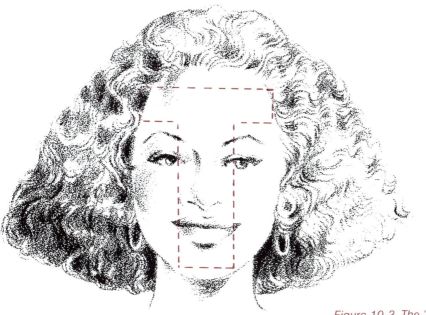

Figure 10-3. The "T" zone area.

101

CARING FOR BLACK SKIN

In spite of the many positive characteristics of Black skin, it should not be taken for granted or neglected. Black clients should be encouraged to have regular professional skin care. Proper care o Black skin enhances its beauty, health, and strength. A healthy, natura glow is priceless.

Because of the abundance of sebum often found in Black skin it should be cleansed thoroughly, and a daily routine using properly balanced products for the individual skin type should be followed Improper diet and lack of daily care can result in an increase in the occurrence of acne, blackheads and pimples.

> *Caution:* Black skin easily suffers change in pigmentation (light and dark spots) due to injury or abrasive handling. For this reason aesthetic treatments such as dermabrasion and exfoliation should be avoided when servicing Black clients. Products that offer a gentle sloughing action may be used, if needed, to remove dead skin cells and rejuvenate the complexion.

Facials

A good way to beautify both oily and dry skin is with a facial Following are two facials that will prove helpful to many of your Black clients. Facials should be performed in the privacy of a booth o room, located in a quiet area. Facial masks for different skin types are available commercially and are of great benefit when applied to the client.

Preparation for a Facial

1. Have the client remove any jewelry and place it safely awa
2. Have the client remove dress, blouse, or sweater and careful hang it up.
3. Wash your hands.
4. Prepare the facial chair by covering it. Then place a clean tow across the back of the facial chair. At no time should the client bare shoulders touch the chair.
5. When seated in the facial chair, remove the client's shoes ar place slippers on the feet.
6. Place a towel over the client's chest. Then pull the cover ov the client. Fold a towel over the cover.
7. Place a towel over the client's hair. There are several types head coverings on the market. Some types are of a turban desig others are designed with elastic, similar to a shower cap (Figure 10-4 through 10-6). They are generally made of either cloth paper towels.
8. Remove lingerie straps from the client's shoulders and adjust th towel, draping it across her chest and the middle of her bac (Alternate method: If the client is given a strapless gown to wea tuck the shoulder lingerie straps into the top of the gown.)

9. Adjust the headrest, then lower the facial chair to a reclining position. A treatment table can also be used when administering facials, especially if a massage will be part of the service.

10. Sanitize hands.

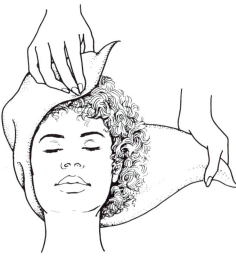

Figure 10-4. Fold the towel lengthwise from one of the top corners to the oppositer lower corner; place it over the headrest with the fold facing down. Place the towel on the headrest before the client enters the facial area. When the client is in a reclining position, the back of the head should rest on the towel so that one side of the towel can be brought up to the center of the forehead to cover the hairline.

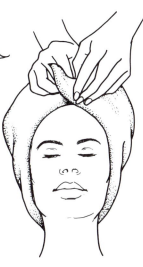

Figure 10-5. With the other hand bring the other side of the towel over the center and cross it over.

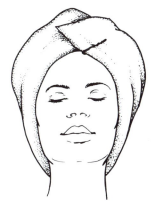

Figure 10-6. Use a regular bobby pin to hold the towel in place. Check to be sure that all strands of hair are tucked under the towel, earlobes are not bent, and the towel is not wrapped too tightly. For paper towel procedure, follow your instructor's guidelines.

*Procedure for a Facial
for Oily Skin and
Blackheads*

1. Apply cleansing cream; remove it with warm cotton pads. If th skin is extremely oily, it may be washed with warm water ar a medicated soap.

2. Apply cleansing lotion.

   a. Remove a little cleansing cream from the jar with a spatul blend cream with the fingers to soften.

   b. Apply cream over the face, using both hands. Start at the chi and with a sweeping motion, spread cream to the end of th jaw, from the base of the nose to the temples, along the sid of the nose, up over the bridge, between the brows, and acros the forehead to the temples (Figure 10-7).

   c. Take additional cream and blend. Smooth down the neck wit long, even strokes.

   d. Starting at the center of the forehead, go lightly around th eyes to the temples and back to the center of the forehead

   e. Slide your fingers down the nose to the upper lip, smooth the temples and forehead, lightly down to the chin, then firm up to the jawline to the temples and forehead.

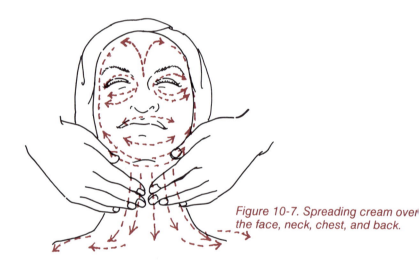

Figure 10-7. Spreading cream over the face, neck, chest, and back.

3. Reapply cleansing cream and steam the face with 3 or 4 mois warm towels or a facial steamer to open the pores.

4. Cover your fingertips with tissues and gently press out ar blackheads. Do not press so hard that you bruise skin tissu Blackheads can also be removed with a sanitized comedor extractor.

5. Sponge the face with antiseptic.

6. Cover the client's eyes with pads moistened with witch hazel (boric acid solution.

7. Apply blue light over the bare skin for not more than 3 to 5 minute

8. Apply a massage cream suitable for this condition.

9. Give facial manipulations.

10. Remove cream with cotton pads.

11. Moisten a cotton pad with an astringent lotion. Apply it to the face and neck with upward and outward motions to close the pores.
12. Blot excess moisture with tissues.
13. Apply foundation and makeup as desired.
14. Return the facial chair to an upright position.
15. Remove the protective head covering.
16. Remove the protective towel and body covering.
17. Assist the client with her clothes and shoes.

Procedure for a Facial for Dry Skin

1. Apply cleansing cream; remove with cotton pads.
2. Sponge the face with cleansing lotion for dry skin.
3. Apply massage cream.
4. Apply lubricating oil or eye cream over and under the eyes.
5. Apply lubricating oil over the neck.
6. Cover the client's eyes with cotton pads moistened with witch hazel or boric acid solution.
7. Expose the face and neck to infrared rays for not more than 5 minutes.
8. Give facial manipulations 3 to 5 times.
9. Remove massage cream and oil with tissues or cotton pads.
10. Apply skin lotion suitable for dry skin.
11. Blot the face with tissues.
12. Apply foundation and makeup as desired.
13. Complete as in a facial for oily skin.

Note: This type of facial may be given with galvanic current to be especially beneficial to dry skin.

SKIN CONDITIONS AFFECTING BLACK SKIN

Several conditions often affect Black skin including: Melasma, vitiligo, pseudofolliculitis, ashiness, and keloids. The cosmetologist should be able to recognize obvious skin conditions as well as diseases and cases of severe acne, eczema, or allergies. The client whose skin is affected by any of these conditions should be advised to see a dermatologist before receiving skin care treatments.

Melasma

Melasma *(mel-**AZ**-ma)* (also known as chloasma) is characterized by dark spots that are usually spread in a band across the middle of the face. This condition is frequently the result of hormonal imbalance associated with pregnancy. Advise any client who appears to have this condition to consult a physician immediately.

Vitiligo

Vitiligo *(vit-i-**LI**-go)* is characterized by white spots on the skin. This condition is caused by the destruction of pigment cells (melanocytes).

Pseudofolliculitis

Pseudofolliculitis *(SOO-doh-foh-lik-u-LI-tis)* is the medical name for ingrown hair. The hair (usually beard hair) curves and reenters the skin, causing infection, which can lead to scarring (Figure 10-8). Cleansing treatments and facial massage will usually help to prevent this condition.

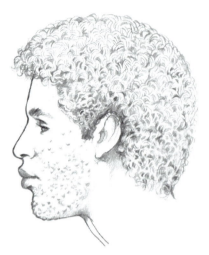

Figure 10-8. Pseudofoliculitis results when the hair tips curve and penetrate the skin just before they would normally exit through the orifice.

Ashiness

Ashiness *(ASH-ee-ness)* is a condition in which the skin becomes gray and flaky in spots (especially on the arms and legs). It is caused by temperature and humidity changes, which cause the skin to quickly lose moisture. Moisturizing creams and lotions are beneficial in relieving this condition.

Keloids

Keloids *(KE-loyds)* are thick scars resulting from the excess growth of fibrous tissue. This is an especially common problem among Black people. Keloids are the skin's reaction to some type of injury or infection. Clients who are prone to keloids should be advised to carefully consider the risks of any cosmetic treatments such as ear piercing or electrology that might cause the condition to erupt. Keloidal clients should be tested on an inconspicuous area of the skin to see if a keloid arises from the esthetic treatment in question.

QUESTIONS FOR REVIEW

1. What is the basic structure of the skin?
2. What are three special characteristics of Black skin?
3. How is a facial for oily skin given?
4. What are three skin conditions affecting Black skin?

Chapter 11 Hair Structure

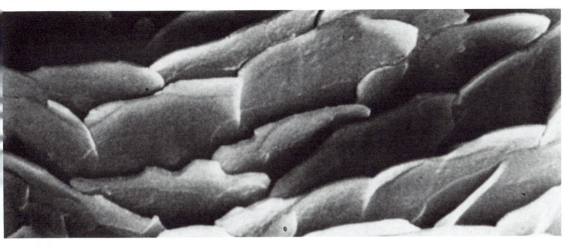

LEARNING OBJECTIVES

After you have mastered this chapter, you will be able to:
1. Define the structure of the hair and explain its function.
2. Describe the characteristics of the cuticle and outline the differences among races.
3. Explain the curl and color configuration in the cortex of Black hair.
4. Describe the structure of the medulla.
5. Explain the importance of varying chemical services on different types of hair.
6. Outline at least three critical differences when permanent waving Black hair.
7. Describe the categories of color available and their effect on Black hair.
8. List types of relaxers available and briefly describe their effect on the hair.

INTRODUCTION

The professional cosmetologist should always understand the medium or fabric upon which they are working, namely hair. By understanding its structure, function, and chemical nature, the stylist can predict the success of each treatment. Problems can be avoided and corrective treatments can be performed with greater confidence.

HAIR STRUCTURE

All hair consists of the protein, **keratin** *(KER-a-tin)*. Keratin is known for its sulfur content, its resistance to being dissolved, and for strength.

The structure of hair is slightly different for varied racial groups. It is important that you understand these differences so that the chemical services you provide will have the same results. By treating various hair types differently you can achieve the results you desire.

Analysis is always important when offering services in the salon. It is very important that you analyze each client. The differences that we will discuss are general, and it is important that you assess the characteristics of your particular client (Figure 11-1).

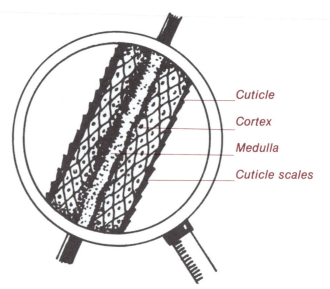

Cuticle

Cortex

Medulla

Cuticle scales

Figure 11-1. Cross section of hair Cuticle

CUTICLE The **cuticle** *(KYOO-ti-kel)* is the outermost layer of the hair. It structure is unique in human hair, and it plays an important pa both to hair that undergoes chemical services and virgin hair, th: is, hair that has not undergone chemical treatment.

Cuticle Characteristics The cuticle consists of overlapping layers (Figure 11-2). Near triangular-shaped cells overlap and wrap around each other so th: its structure resembles a very tiny palm tree trunk. This overlappin structure gives hair much of its pliability, one-fourth of its strengt! and all of its resistance to or absorption of liquids, which is terme _porosity._

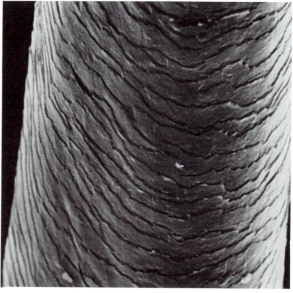

Figure 11-2. The overlapping layers of the cuticle.

Courtesy of Gillette Company Research, Rockville, Md.

108

The cuticle is responsible for the sheen of the hair, and different racial groups show differences in this regard. A flat, compact cuticle will reflect light back to the eye, seen as sheen. Curly hair, having a rougher surface, will show less shine.

There are several schools of thought regarding the cuticle and various racial groups. One holds that different races have varying amounts of cuticle layers: Caucasians have four to seven layers, Blacks have eight to twelve layers, and Orientals have twelve or more. Another theory is that the cuticle layers are compacted as the hair hardens in the follicle, meaning that curly hair has an uneven cuticle with the layers compacted in the curves of a curl formation and smoothed on the outside (see illustration). In either case, there are differences to be considered when performing services on different textures of hair. Most Black hair is resistant to penetration by liquids. This means that the stylist must either use a formulation designed for this resistant hair or allow more time for traditional chemicals to work. It also means that the cuticle will need extra care after treatment through conditioning.

CORTEX   The second layer of the hair is the **cortex** *(KOR-teks)* (Figure 11-3). This layer consists of interwoven fibers arranged in a helix configuration.

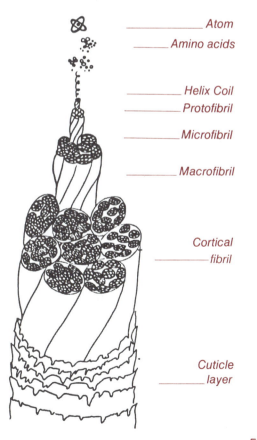

_____ Atom

_____ Amino acids

_____ Helix Coil

_____ Protofibril

_____ Microfibril

_____ Macrofibril

Cortical
_____ fibril

Cuticle
_____ layer

Figure 11-3 Helix configuration of the cortex

Cortex Structure   Fibers wrap around each other in a coil, which then wraps around other coils, and so on, until the total cortex structure can be compared to yarn or rope. This characteristic of the hair makes it extremely strong (Figure 11-4). The hair is able to withstand seven times the weight that a copper wire of exactly the same diameter could hold without breaking. The cortex is responsible for the primary functions of the hair, such as 75 percent of its strength, all of its moisture, elasticity, curl, and nearly all of its color content. The resiliency (resistance to compression) of the hair is also attributed to the cortex.

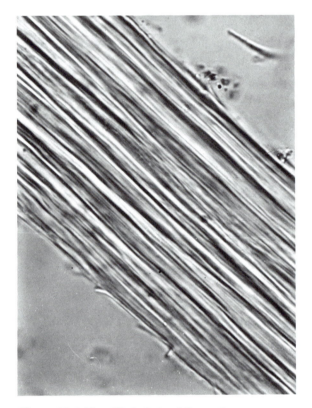

Figure 11-4 Magnified photo of the cortex

Courtesy of Gillette Company Research, Rockville, Md.

The cortex of hair of different racial groups also varies. Black people have a smaller cortex, much like finer textures of hair; Caucasians have a medium texture; and Orientals have a larger diameter of cortex.

In the case of Black hair, these differences must be taken into consideration before giving a chemical service. A finer cortex diameter, for instance, means that the product will act faster once it has penetrated the cuticle and can cause damage if left to process for too long.

A smaller cortex also means that the hair is more susceptible to heat damage. As thermal pressing and styling are prevalent, this means that more reconstructive conditioning is necessary when treating any fine hair type.

Orientals and Blacks have more pigment distributed in the cuticle and, in the case of Orientals, the medulla. Black people have a lower sulfur content, a slightly lower lipid (oil) content, and a sulfur bond that has a different configuration. There are fewer pigment molecules present, although the size of each pigment granule is larger (Figure 11-5).

Various types of pigment granules

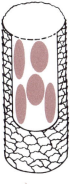 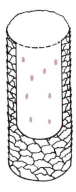 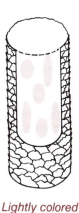

Large　　　　　*Small*　　　　　*Lightly colored*

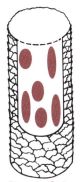 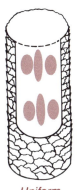 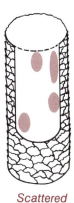

Deeply Colored　　　*Uniform*　　　*Scattered*

Figure 11-5 Various types of pigment granules

Color Pigment

The pigment of Black hair reacts to coloring agents differently. Because it has a larger molecular structure, it will react more quickly to lightening and can result in a *brassy* appearance. Black and red natural pigment will quickly oxidize to the red gold or gold stage because of the higher concentration of red pigmentation. Because of this, different formulations should be mixed when lightening. It is often difficult to lift the hair above the gold stage, however, because the pigment molecules are almost exclusively melanin in very dark hair. The additional activators, time, and sometimes heat that are required to lift the hair above this stage can cause severe damage.

Coloring products for this type of hair should be able to penetrate quickly and should be carefully monitored by the practitioner to ensure good results. Most formulas should contain drabbers to offset the red or orange result and different volumes of peroxide, such as 25 volume or 30 volume, usually give better results. Another category of hair coloring, semi-permanent tints, are also used extensively, especially those of the translucent type.

Natural Curl Formation

The formation of the sulfur bond determines the curl present in any hair type (Figure 11-6). In the case of Black hair, the bond structure is slanted at a sharp angle, creating various degrees of curl. The sharper the angle, the stronger the curl pattern that is evident.

Several theories attempt to explain the formation of natural curl.

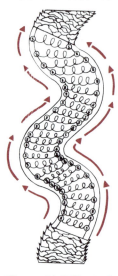

Figure 11-6 Slanted sulfur bond structure of black hair

Shape of the Hair

One of the first theories to be developed was that the shape of the hair was different, depending upon the curl present. Although there are definite differences in the hair shape of various racial groups, it does not seem to be dependent upon natural curl.

Most Oriental people, for example, have a structure that is known as **quadlobular** *(kwad-LOH-byoo-lar)*. When this hair is examined under a microscope, four lobes can usually be seen. The overall shape of the hair is round, or sometimes nearly square (Figure 11-7).

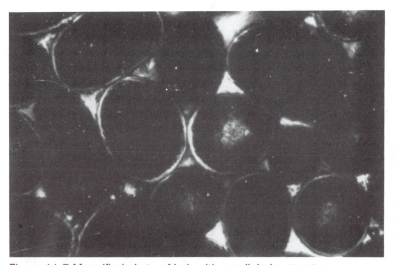

Figure 11-7 Magnified photo of hair with quadlobular structure
Courtesy of Gillette Company Research, Rockville, Md.

112

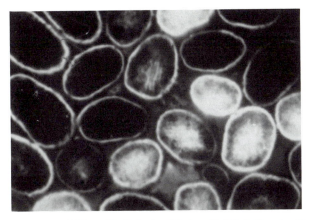

*Figure 11-8 Magnified photo of hair with trilobular structure
Courtesy of Gillette Company Research, Rockville, Md.*

Most Caucasian people have a hair structure that has a **trilobular** *(treye-**LOH**-byoo-lar)* shape. Three lobes can be seen under a microscope, and the overall shape is an oval (Figure 11-8).

Most Black people have a hair shape that is **bilobular** *(beye-**LOH**-byoo-lar)*. Under a microscope, two lobes can generally be seen, and the overall shape is flat (Figure 11-9).

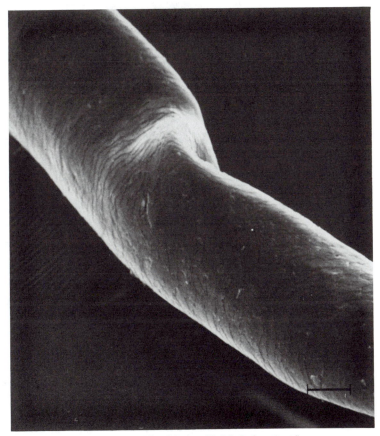

*Figure 11-9 Magnified photo of hair with bilobular structure
Courtesy of Gillette Company Research, Rockville, Md.*

Shape of the Follicle

Another school of thought was that the shape of the follic[le] determined the shape of the forming hair. A round, straight follic[le] produced straight hair; an oval, slightly curved follicle produced wave[y] hair; and a flat, distorted follicle produced curly hair.

We now know that this theory is incorrect. The soft keratin of th[e] follicle takes on the shape of the hair within it. We also know th[at] all follicles surrounding an **anagen (AN**-ah-jen) or forming hair, ar[e] straight. **Catagen (CAT**-ah-jen), or resting hair, begins to assum[e] the shape of the hair, and often curves if the hair is curly. The follic[le] surrounding a **telogen (TEL**-oh-jen) hair is shorter, club-shaped a[t] the bottom, and often distorted if the hair is curly.

Cyclical Theory

Biochemists propose a theory that the curl of the hair is determine[d] by the **germinal matrix (JUR**-mi-nal **MAY**-triks). (Figure 11-10).

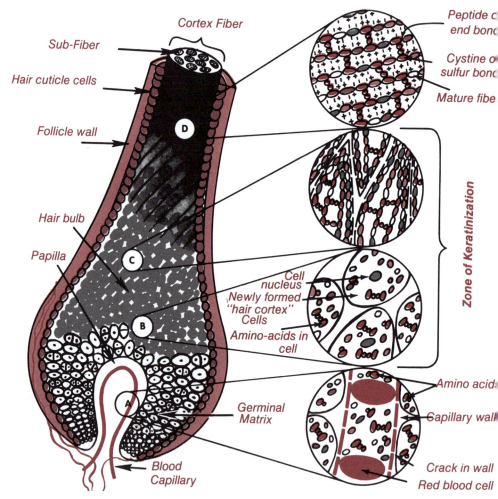

Figure 11-10 Germinal matrix

This specialized group of cells has an uneven rate of cell division first on one side of the germinal matrix, then on the other side. The end result is that the bonding structure of the hair is uneven. The disulfide bond, responsible for curl, forms at an angle. The sharper the angle, the stronger the curl pattern evident to the eye. It is generally assumed that genetic factors control the germinal matrix.

MEDULLA   It was once thought that not all hair types contained a medulla, or an innermost layer. We now know that all hair contains a medulla during its formation, but that due to its fragile construction, the medulla can be destroyed by both chemical and physical services performed.

The medulla is a loose arrangement of cells, much resembling a natural sponge. The content of the medulla in the hair is very small, 2 to 5 percent, and can be easily compacted by physical services such as thermal styling or by the swelling of the cortex during chemical services.

The function of the medulla has never been proven, but it is thought to excrete materials from the hair as well as serving as a source for moisture and nutrients. If the medulla is destroyed, the hair might break during combing, styling, or chemical services.

CHEMICAL SERVICES   The best way to ensure good results on various textures of hair is to analyze the hair and carefully consider the manner in which it will react to the chemicals applied. We will discuss here the differences to consider for certain clients or for certain types of hair. You will find the step-by-step procedure for each service in that particular chapter.

PERMANENT WAVES   The intent of permanent waving is always to alter the natural curl present. For most Caucasians, this means adding curl. For most ethnic people, it means reducing the curl and making the hair more manageable by the conventional means of setting, blow-drying, and air-drying.

Permanent waving to reduce curl present is known as soft curl permanent waving because the original technique created soft curls that could be air dried. Soft curls are used today to create a variety of effects. The only limitations to the process are these:

- Soft curls may NOT be given on hair treated with sodium hydroxide. In your analysis determine what services the client has received on the hair and also inquire about retail products used at home because some shampoos and conditioners also contain sodium hydroxide. Soft curl lotion contains ammonium thioglycolate, which is not compatible with sodium hydroxide. If the hair has been relaxed, disulfide bonds have been chemically altered into lanthionine bonds. This is a permanent chemical reaction that cannot be reversed. At the very least, you will not achieve the desired curl pattern; at the worst, the hair will dissolve due to the reaction of the chemicals.

- Soft curls cannot safely remove all the curl from the hair. If your client wants very smooth, nearly straight hair, you will get better results with a regular relaxing process.

Wrapping with Control   The first consideration is the curl pattern itself. If the natural pattern is strong or tight, a prewrap solution will be necessary. This solution, which opens the cuticle and begins the process of breaking the sulfur bonds, helps the stylist control the hair while wrapping. It begins the process of softening and swelling the hair, making it more pliable. Most of the solutions are thick so that the weight will temporarily straighten the natural curl. They also contain **surfactants** *(sur-FAK-tants),* ingredients to reduce the resistance of the cuticle surface to lotion penetration (Figure 11-11).

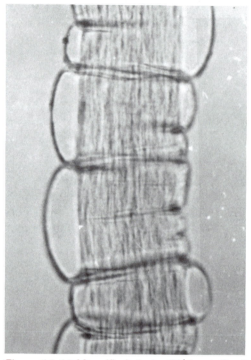

Figure 11-11 Magnified photo of hair swollen by pre-wrap solution

As with any perm, the quality of the wrap will determine the quality of the finished wave. The change in the hair is more evident after a soft curl, however, so the details of a good wrap are even more apparent. Each subsection should be no larger than the length and diameter of the rod; slightly smaller subsections give better curl and results on very thick or excessively curly hair. When the wrap is completed, the rods should be nearly touching. Too much tension can break the hair, but slightly more stress is needed during the wrap to reduce the natural curl. Due to the cortex, the hair is often more fragile during the processing time. Great care should be used so that the bands of the rods do not compress the hair, which will result in breakage. Many stylists prefer the double-flat, or two-end paper wrap to further protect the ends if they are frayed or if the hair has been thermal pressed.

Processing Factors

Carefully analyze the porosity of the hair. Due to the cuticle structure, select a processing lotion that will penetrate faster or allow more time for this phase of the service. Lotions also contain surfactants and are usually thicker—a gel or cream, for example—so that the lotion will adhere to the hair and will not dry as rapidly.

As the lotion penetrates, the stylist will notice that the sheen of the hair increases. As the cuticle layer swells, the hair reflects more light. This is an indication that the lotion is entering the cortex and that careful checking of the processing should begin.

Once the lotion has entered the cortex, the processing time is usually rapid. Most Black hair has less cortex, so there are fewer disulfide links to be broken. To take a test curl, first gently blot the rods with a damp terry towel or dry paper towel. This removes excess lotion so that the curl's true development can be seen. The thickness of the lotion might otherwise cause a false test curl. The natural curl pattern of the hair will first expand, or straighten, then the hair will begin to conform to the size of the rod. The hair must be long enough to encircle the rod at least 2-1/2 times, and the rod size should be at least two sizes larger than the natural curl for visible results from the soft curl process.

Once the curl pattern is desirable, remove lotion from the hair by blotting or rinsing as directed by the manufacturer.

Special Considerations

This is an ideal time to strengthen the cortex of fragile hair by conditioning. Lightly spray a penetrating conditioner over the rods. It is important not to oversaturate the hair and prevent good neutralization. This technique is especially good if the hair has previously been thermal pressed or if a retouch curl is being given.

After the hair has been neutralized according to the manufacturer's directions, the stylist should consider the best way to acidify the hair. After any chemical service, the hair should be acidified to help close the cuticle and begin the hair's return to its acid state. Naturally excessively curly hair, however, can have a tendency to *revert* or become too curly again if the acidification solution is too strong. Most manufacturers recommend that the stylist apply a cream moisturizer that is acid balanced between 4.5 and 5.5. This will smooth the cuticle, which is roughened due to the penetration process, and slowly begin acidification. As with any chemical service, care should be taken when removing tangles and less heat and stretching should be used to achieve the desired style. Ideally the hair should air dry or be wet set; however, popular styles cannot always be created in this fashion. Thermal styling can be done as long as the practitioner considers the state of the hair and protects it with a styling lotion.

A unique situation that can occur with the soft curl process is the need to reduce the curl of the new growth without damaging the previously permed hair. This is commonly called a recurl. The soft curl process gives the client the option of longer styles without the excessive damage that pressing would cause. As a result, the client might return and request that the regrowth be soft curled with as little hair trimmed as possible.

It is best to use a *two step* product for the recurl because you will have the ability to presoften only the curly regrowth. After the hair is sufficiently softened, you can proceed with the wrap after applying a cream conditioner to the previously treated hair, or you can do any of the "root perm" techniques. The hair should be lightly conditioned after processing, and you might prefer to use partial or complete air oxidation during the neutralizing phase. It is important that the recurl be performed with a product compatible with the original soft curl.

HAIR COLORING   Present day hair coloring products offer many choices for the Black client. Due to the amount of color that is present in the skin and hair, many shades can be created and fad and avant garde techniques can be stunning. We will not discuss any specific trends here, but will instead outline the method to approach hair coloring for Black clients so that you can make the choices appropriate for your client.

Temporary Color   Temporary color will deposit, but will not lift. Today's gels and mousses are an excellent way to add highlights, increase sheen, or create special effects. Use color theory to determine what the result will be for the color you are adding. The addition of red-based and blue-based colors usually yields the most popular and richest results. Because of the resistant porosity and the usually darker pigment present, temporary colors that are combined with styling aids are the most effective.

Semi-Permanent Colors   This entire class of coloring products can be very effective and exciting for the Black client. As the stylist, you will take advantage of the color already present in the hair and skin.

Translucent colors can be used to add outstanding sheen and warm tones for fashion effects. Translucent colors are available from many manufacturers and can be used with or without heat. Results are deeper and longer lasting as heat is used, depending upon the porosity of the hair.

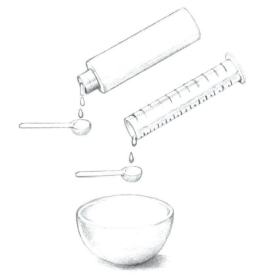

Stains, that is, permanent tints that are mixed with penetrating conditioner rather than peroxide, can add all the auburns and rich browns (Figure 11-12). Dramatic effects can be achieved with a blue-black, or you can correct lightening caused by chemicals, heat, and sun exposure without further damaging the hair. These effects last from 4 to 8 weeks, depending upon the porosity of the hair. Best results are achieved by placing a plastic cap over the hair and processing under heat for 15 to 30 minutes. If you are using a stain for corrective color, try adding a small amount such as 1/2 ounce of 5 percent peroxide.

Permanent Tints   This category of color causes a chemical reaction within the cortex of the hair. For that reason, the colorist should carefully analyze any client's hair and skin (Figure 11-13).

Factors to consider are:

- **Skin tones.** What are the undertones of the client? What base colors would enhance the natural facial tone? What contrast would the client like to see, or with what change will he or she feel comfortable? What is the life-style of the individual, and how much time is he or she prepared to take to care for permanently colored hair?

- **Porosity.** What is the porosity of the hair? If it is resistant you will have to vary your formulation with slightly higher volumes of peroxide. If it is damaged from chemical or heat exposure, you will have to lower the volume to prevent further damage, excess lightening, or patchy results.

- **Condition.** Consider the entire hair strand. If the ends have been relaxed or thermal pressed, you might have to alter your formula. If the hair is long enough to have had several chemical processes, consider the use of a stain on the ends and regular color near the base. Another technique is to lower the volume by diluting with shampoo, conditioner, or distilled water as you apply from the scalp area outward.

Tint and conditioning mix

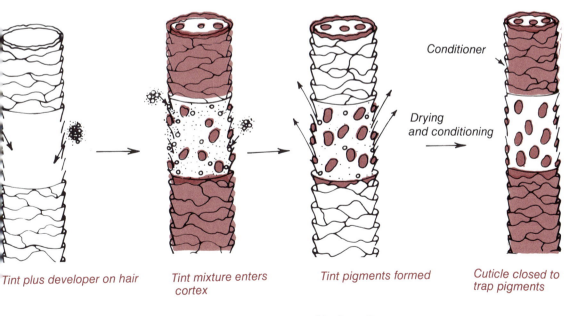

| Tint plus developer on hair | Tint mixture enters cortex | Tint pigments formed | Cuticle closed to trap pigments |

Conditioner

Drying and conditioning

Figure 11-13 Tint and conditioning mix

- **Lightening.** If you intend to lighten the hair you must conside two things: the resistance of the cuticle to penetration and the larger pigment molecule present in the cortex. Initially, the hai will be slow to process, but once the color has penetrated you will have to contend with *brassy* shades of red, red-gold and gold (Figure 11-14). Additive colors or formulations with more drabbers will help you overcome this if it is not a desired effect. Again, slightly higher volumes of peroxide are usually more effective if you are lightening the hair. Application or damp, clean hair will improve absorption of the color.

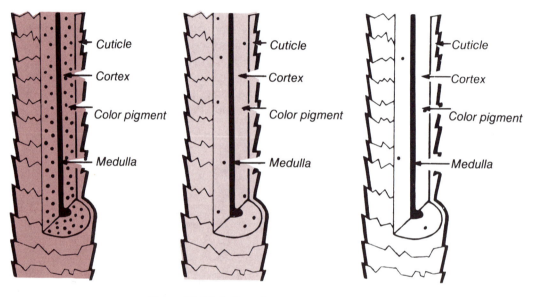

Figure 11-14 Action of permanent tints on hair

- **Deposit.** If you want to deposit color but do not want the lifting action of a one-step tint to show, lower the volume of peroxide to 10 or use tint formulations without ammonia that have no lifting capabilities. Remember that the hair will be more prone to fading over time due to its pigment molecule size.
- **Irritation.** The scalp of your Black client may be more dry than the scalp of other clients. Be sure to check for scalp abrasions and irritations and always perform a patch test 24 hours prior to the color application.
- **Elasticity.** If the hair has been processed before, including pressing services, elasticity is reduced. The hair contains fewer salt and hydrogen bonds, which provide elasticity, and all curl reduction services require some pressure on the hair. Use a tint brush or applicator bottle and work the formula gently through the hair with the fingers, never a comb.

● **Coatings.** If coating agents have been used in shampoos, conditioners, or activators, a buildup will be present on the hair. This will prevent penetration of the color formula, uneven results, and excessive dryness and brittleness in the hair. Retail appropriate home care items. If the condition is extreme, remove the coating agents, deep-condition the hair, and postpone the service until a later date.

Special Considerations

Hair that has been relaxed has greater porosity. The advanced technician can take advantage of this condition and create many coloring effects that will last longer on the hair.

If the hair fades or if you have more warm tones than you desire, consider using a staining technique. You can add the necessary color, blue for example, and correct the condition without deepening the color.

Aftercare

Acidification is also important, as in every chemical service. Precautions must again be taken not to overacidify and cause curl reversion or a brittle condition in the cuticle.

The hair should be moisturized, and the client should always use an instant conditioner after shampooing. The cuticle will need smoothing for good styling results and protection with a styling aid.

RELAXERS

There are many types of relaxers available to today's technician. You should select the appropriate one based upon your analysis of the client's hair texture, condition, porosity, natural curl, and desired style.

Relaxers are divided into two categories based upon the activity of their primary ingredients.

Thio Relaxers

Ammonium thioglycolate, the primary ingredient of permanent waves, can be used as a relaxing product. This type of relaxer is often chosen if the hair is fine or if the client does not want all of the curl removed.

Cream or gel formulas are used, however, so that the weight of the solution will assist in the reduction of the curl. Many stylists actually use the soft curl products and eliminate the use of rods. The hair can be neutralized in the straightened position, or it can be molded, sculpted, or waved. Many technicians neutralize the hair through a net to keep it in place.

Analysis of the client's scalp is always important because the product might touch the scalp during the process. Use special care, a protective cream around the hairline and over the ears, and gently blot any product from the scalp.

Thio relaxers work by penetrating through the cuticle layer and breaking the disulfide linkage (Figure 11-15). The hair is then manipulated into the desired state of smoothness before neutralizing. The neutralizer is actually an oxidizing formula, usually hydrogen peroxide or sodium bromate, that will combine with the excess hydrogen introduced by the lotion. The result is the reformation of the disulfide bond in the new configuration.

Figure 11-15. Chemical hair straightening with ammonium thioglycolate

1. Virgin curly hair
Virgin polypeptide chains show original position of cystine disulfide links between them.

2. Processing
Reduced S-bonds (breaking the cystine disulfide links)

3. Neutralizing
Prepared neutralizer poured through hair, after smoothing and straightening.

4 Rinsing
Excess neutralizer and water removed leaving hair in a straightened position.

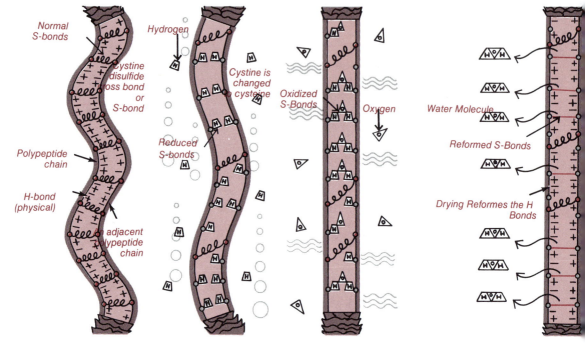

Normal S-bonds

Hydrogen

Cystine disulfide cross bond or S-bond

Cystine is changed to cystine

Oxidized S-Bonds

Oxygen

Water Molecule

Polypeptide chain

Reduced S-bonds

Reformed S-Bonds

H-bond (physical)

Drying Reformes the H Bonds

An adjacent polypeptide chain

Sodium Hydroxide Relaxers

This category of relaxers has expanded in recent years to include cream relaxers whose primary active ingredient is sodium hydroxide or any of several similar agents, calcium hydroxide, and so on.

These relaxers are used more often than the thio type because they are much faster in their action, can remove more curl from the hair, do not require damaging physical manipulation to reduce the curl, and last far longer.

As the technician, always carefully consider which type of relaxer to use. Sodium and thio relaxer types are NOT interchangeable so the client will have to continue with the same product category or let the hair regrow until all the formerly processed hair has been removed by cutting before switching products.

Action of Sodium Hydroxide Relaxers

The cream first penetrates the cuticle. The disulfide bond is then broken, and the weight of the cream physically shifts the position of the polypeptide chains (Figure 11-16). Hair should be relaxed only 75 to 80 percent, no more.

Rinsing the hair with warm water to thoroughly remove the relaxer stops the processing. This is an extremely important step. The water should be warm, but not hot. Hot water could damage the hair, cause scalp irritation, and be extremely uncomfortable for the client. Rinsing should be thorough, starting with moderate water pressure and gradually increasing it to help remove excess cream from the hair

Figure 11-16. **Chemical Hair Straightening—Sodium Hydroxide**

1. Curly Hair
Both H and S bonds holding polypeptide chains in position.

2 Hair Being Processed
All H-bonds broken, most S-bonds broken. Hand and comb manipulations starting to relax wave. (Polypeptide chains shift.)

3. Hair Being Neutralized
The neutralizer fixes polypeptide chains in a straigh position after hair has been fully relaxed.

4. Straighetened hair
After rinsing and proper drying. Lanthionine cross links now exist between polypeptide chains, keeping the hair in a permanently straight form. Drying reforms the physical bonds.

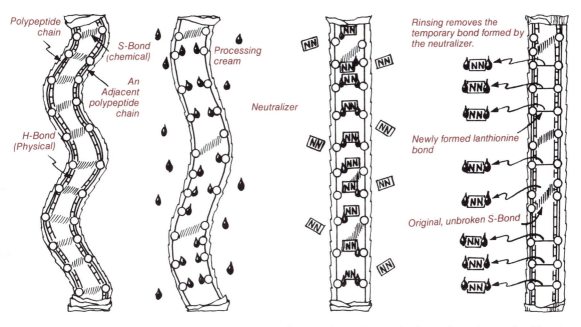

Polypeptide chain
S-Bond (chemical)
An Adjacent polypeptide chain
H-Bond (Physical)
Processing cream
Neutralizer
Rinsing removes the temporary bond formed by the neutralizer.
Newly formed lanthionine bond
Original, unbroken S-Bond

Direct the stream of water from the scalp through to the ends. Check the back and nape area carefully and lift the client's head slightly to ensure thorough rinsing. Continue until the water runs clear and you no longer see foam.

The next chemical phase is the shampoo. An acid is needed to react with the chemical still remaining in the hair. A common way to accomplish this is to shampoo the hair thoroughly with an acid-balanced shampoo. Many manufacturers offer products known as neutralizing shampoos for this purpose. You should check to ensure that the product offered has an acidic pH between 4.5 and 5.5.

You will notice a sulfur-like smell on the hair during the shampoo. This is evidence of the desired chemical neutralization occurring. Rinse and reapply shampoo until the hair foams well, then rinse again.

This acidification is all that is necessary to neutralize the chemicals still remaining in the hair. Oxidizer solutions should NOT be used because they will only damage the hair. The chemical activity forms a completely new bond, lanthionine *(LAN-thio-neen)* in the hair.

Lanthionine cannot be reduced or oxidized. This process is permanent and cannot be reversed. As a result a chemical product that contains thio will not only be ineffective on this hair type, it can also cause severe damage.

There are many ways that the experienced technician can customize the relaxer service according to the analysis of the client's hair and the style desired.

If the hair is fine, has been tinted, or has areas of damage, conditioning is necessary. If the damage is severe, postpone the relaxer service until a series of deep-penetrating conditioning treatments are given.

If the damage is minor or if you wish to protect the already processed hair during a retouch application, apply a cream penetrating conditioner to the processed ends. Continue with your service, being careful not to overlap the relaxer on previously relaxed hair.

Another option you may choose is to neutralize the relaxer residue inside the cortex with a conditioner rather than with a shampoo after processing. Apply conditioner as you would a shampoo (use slightly more product) and massage gently through the hair. Leave on for 2 to 5 minutes, depending on the penetration ability of the product chosen, and rinse. Repeat with a second application. Massage the second application through the hair. You will have a very slight foaming action. Time again and rinse. This technique both neutralizes the chemical and conditions the hair at a point when the cuticle is open and the hair very receptive. You will notice a marked improvement on retouched hair, especially if it tends to be dry or brittle. This is also excellent for fine hair; however, you may have some difficulty with styling because fine hair becomes very soft and silky.

Regardless of the techniques chosen, all relaxed hair should be conditioned at some point during the service. The most common choice is after the shampoo. The hair should always be styled with a heat protective styling agent.

Relaxing is probably the only chemical service in which it is important that the hair NOT be preshampooed. Scalp irritation is always a concern, and shampooing prior to the service could cause irritation that would force you to remove the relaxing cream before processing is complete. Advise your client against brushing the hair the day of the service and caution him or her not to shampoo for at least 24 hours prior to the appointment. If you determine that there is an excessive buildup of pressing aids, activators, or other coating agents that requires removing, remove the buildup and condition but postpone the service.

Protective Bases

Protective creams, once known as *bases* still have their place in today's salon. Every client should have protective cream around the hairline, over the ears, and around the face. Some technicians feel more secure if they use a base during a virgin application since they have no way of knowing the client's sensitivity level. And some technicians still prefer to use a relaxer product that requires a base, especially on excessively curly, resistant hair.

A base can be any product that either has a pH balance low enough to counter the caustic pH of the relaxer (lower than 4.5) or contains petrolatum that will prevent the penetration of the relaxer into the skin. In either case, the cream should be resistant to dissolving in water. The stylist should still carefully blot any relaxer that contacts the base.

No-base relaxers are slightly milder in their action and contain agents that are designed to protect the scalp during application. Protective base should still be used around the hairline.

Aftercare   As with any chemical service, the client should return home with a supply of quality shampoo and conditioner to maintain the hair's condition. The curl reduction with a relaxer can be quite drastic, so spend time teaching your client which method of styling is best for the style selected and be sure to include styling aids in the retail package. Schedule conditioning treatments between retouch applications or other chemical services.

With today's chemical products, it is quite safe to thermal style relaxed hair as long as good techniques and products are used. Caution your clients about the use of excessive heat, however. Also show them how to achieve the style they want without stretching the hair excessively. The hair should NOT be thermal pressed, nor should the client use (and especially sleep in) sponge rollers. Both cause too much compression of the hair, which results in breakage. Pressing can also discolor the hair, especially if it is light, lightened, or gray. It is highly unusual to have a relaxer client that has a double-processed coloring service. If this should happen, thermal styling of any type is not recommended.

Contrary to some client's opinions, the hair can be shampooed as often as necessary. There will be no adverse results as long as good quality products are used for maintenance. Shampooing will not cause faster regrowth, reversion, or loss of hair. On the other hand, the buildup caused by old-fashioned styling agents or repeated styling without shampooing will cause dryness, brittleness, and can result in unbecoming styles and breakage.

By understanding the hair, its structures and functions, the professional cosmetologist can predict the success of each treatment. Problems can be avoided, and corrective treatments can be performed with greater confidence. The stylist can then be more competitive in the salon, giving better services with greater value.

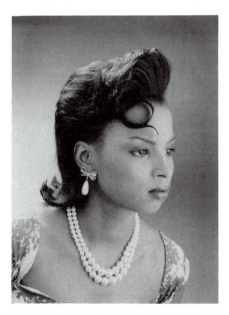

1. What is the structure of the hair and what is its function?
2. What are the characteristics of the cuticle and how does it differ among races?
3. How is the curl and color configured in the cortex of Black hair?
4. How is the medulla structured?
5. Why is it important to vary chemical services on different types of hair?
6. What are three critical differences when permanent waving Black hair?
7. What are the categories of color available and what are their effects on Black hair?
8. What types of relaxers are available? How do they affect the hair?

Chapter 12 Hair Coloring

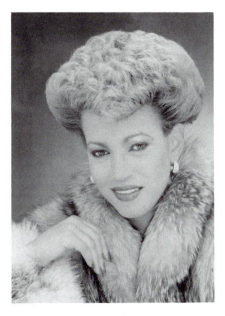

LEARNING OBJECTIVES

After you have mastered this chapter, you will be able to:

1. List five reasons for coloring or lightening hair.
2. Give the three classifications of hair coloring.
3. Explain how pigment molecules in Black hair are different from pigment molecules in Caucasian hair.
4. Give the procedure for an aniline derivative tint patch test.
5. List the basic rules of color selection.
6. Explain what volumes of peroxide most colorists prefer when working with Black hair.
7. List the advantages and disadvantages of temporary hair colorings.
8. Explain the procedure for semi-permanent hair coloring.
9. Give the procedure for a single-process tint.
10. Give the procedure for a single-process tint retouch.
11. Explain how highlighting shampoo tints are prepared.
12. Tell what pre-softening does.
13. Give five tips and safety precautions for coloring Black hair.
14. Give twelve general safety precautions for coloring and lightening.

INTRODUCTION

Hair coloring (tinting) is the science and art of changing the color of hair. Hair coloring involves the addition of an artificial color to the natural pigment in the hair, the lightening of natural pigment, or the addition of color to lightened hair. (The terms *tinting* and *coloring* are used interchangeably in this text.)

THE COLORING SERVICE

Skill in hair coloring and lightening can be accomplished by continuous practice and study. They can become profitable sources of income in the salon because they represent repeat business. The client who has tinted hair usually returns to the salon for retouching at regular intervals. Satisfactory service will encourage a return to the same salon

The principal reasons for coloring or lightening hair are as follows:

1. Restore gray hair to its natural shade
2. Change the natural shade of hair to a more attractive color
3. Restore hair to its natural color
4. Create decorative effects
5. Enhance or create highlights

Typical clients include the following:

1. People with prematurely gray hair
2. Business people who think that the shade of their hair is a handicap
3. People who want to maintain a youthful appearance
4. People who want to refine and enhance their color tones for fashion purposes

The successful cosmetologist must know the following:

1. Structure of the hair and scalp
2. Proper selection and application of coloring and lightening products
3. Chemical reactions of tints and lighteners

> **Note:** Color theory is an important part of proper hair coloring. See chapter 14 for an in-depth explanation of color theory

CLASSIFICATIONS OF HAIR COLORING

Hair coloring is the application of artificial color to the hair. Hair coloring falls into three main categories: **Temporary, semi-permanent**, and **permanent**. The professional colorist must know how each group acts on the hair and also know how hair porosity and the addition of heat affects each category of hair color.

Temporary Hair Coloring

Temporary hair colorings are designed to last on the hair from shampoo to shampoo. Excessively porous hair can cause this type of hair coloring to last longer and fade with each shampoo. A patch test is usually not necessary for this type of hair color. Consult the manufacturer's directions. Temporary color can only deposit pigment, it cannot lift (Figure 12-1).

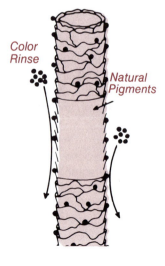

Figure 12-1.
Water or Color Rinses

Color Rinse

Natural Pigments

1. Color rinses are prepared rinses used either to highlight or add color to the hair. They contain certified colors and remain on the hair until the next shampoo.
2. Highlighting color shampoos combine the action of a color rinse with that of a shampoo. These shampoos give highlights and add color tones to the hair.
3. Crayons and mascara are temporary colors used to add color to the eyebrows and lashes.
4. Hair color sprays are applied to dry hair from aerosol containers for special or party effects.

Semi-permanent Hair Coloring   Semi-permanent hair coloring agents are formulated to last from four to six shampoos. They penetrate into the cuticle layer and on over-porous hair can penetrate into the cortex for a more permanent effect. They are applied without peroxide, so they do not change the basic structure of the hair. The addition of heat, however, can sometimes make this type of hair color much more lasting. Be guided by the information supplied by the manufacturer and your instructor's directions.

Semi-permanent colors are designed to add color to the hair (Figure 12-2). They can be used in the following ways:

Semi-Permanent Color

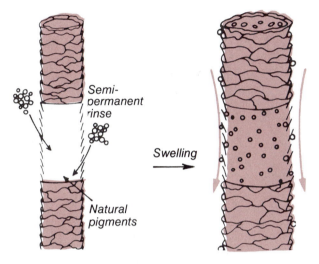

Figure 12-2. Semi-permanent color penetrates the cuticle slightly. Molecules are gradually shampooed from the hair.

1. Cover or blend partially gray hair without affecting its natural color. Most semi-permanent colors are designed to add color to the hair that is 25 percent or less gray.
2. Enhance or blend partially gray hair without affecting its natural color. This can be done successfully on almost any percentage of gray, depending upon the desired color.
3. Highlight and enhance the color tones of the hair. Semi-permanent colors can be used to add golden or red highlights and to deepen the color of the hair. This type of color is especially effective for the Black client.
4. Serve as a non-peroxide toner for pre-lightened hair. Due to the porosity of the hair, the toner will penetrate.

Most semi-permanent hair colors require a patch test, because most contain aniline derivative agents. The following illustrations indicate how this type of hair coloring works on the hair shaft.

Permanent Hair Coloring

Permanent hair colorings are designed to penetrate the cuticle and deposit molecules into the cortex. Due to the penetration and the addition of peroxide, these colors can both lift and deposit (Figure 12-3).

Figure 12-3. Action of hair tints

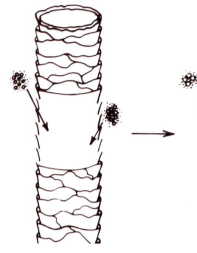
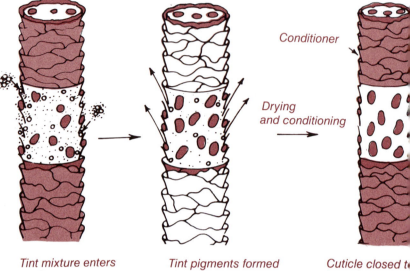

Tint plus developer on hair

Tint mixture enters cortex

Tint pigments formed

Cuticle closed to trap pigments

Conditioner

Drying and conditioning

Aniline derivative tints. These are also known as penetrating tints, synthetic organic tints or oxidation tints, and are commonly called *tints* in the industry. Tints can both lift and deposit and have the widest variety of colors available. Toners also fit in the category of aniline derivative tints but can only deposit tones to pre-lightened hair. A patch test is required for all permanent color that is analine derivative based.

Pure vegetable tints. These have been in use for centuries. In the past, indigo, camomile, sage, and Egyptian henna were used for hair coloring. They deposited a coating on the hair. Today, only henna is still used professionally, although other ingredients are added to it to produce non-red shades. It is important that the person receiving vegetable tints is not also going to undergo a chemical service, because current vegetable products not only coat the hair, but also penetrate. They can prevent absorption of chemicals and cause uneven results, damage, and even breakage.

Metallic or mineral dyes. Dyes such as lead acetate or silver nitrate are the progressive type known as color restorers. They form a metallic coating over the hair shaft, making it unsatisfactory for chemical processing, hair lightening, or tinting. Successive applications are made until the proper shade has developed.

> *Caution:* Metallic dyes are not professional colors and should be avoided.

Compound dyes. These are dyes such as compound henna or combinations of vegetable dyes with certain metallic salts and other dyestuffs. The metallic salts fix the color. Compound dyes coat the hair shaft and make the hair unfit for chemical processing. They are also not used professionally.

Although metallic and compound dyes are never used professionally, people do apply such products to their hair at home. Therefore, the hair colorist must be able to recognize and understand the effects. Such coloring agents must be removed and the hair reconditioned prior to any other chemical service.

Hair treated with metallic or any other coating dye appears to be dry and dull. It is generally harsh and brittle to the touch. These colorings usually fade to unnatural tones. Silver dyes have a greenish cast, lead a purple color, and those containing copper turn a brassy red.

Test for Metallic Salts and Coating Dyes

1. In a glass container, mix 1 ounce of 20-volume (6 percent) peroxide and 20 drops of ammonia.

2. Cut a strand of the client's hair, bind with tape, and immerse it in the solution for 30 minutes.

3. Remove, dry, and observe the strand.

Hair dyed with lead will lighten immediately.

Hair treated with silver will have no reaction at all. This indicates that other chemicals will not be successful because they cannot penetrate the coating.

Hair treated with copper will start to boil and easily pull apart. This hair would be severely damaged or destroyed if other chemicals were applied.

Hair treated with a coating dye will either not change color or will lighten in spots. This hair will not receive chemical services evenly, and the length of time necessary for penetration may damage it.

Specialized shampoos, preparations designed to remove metallics, and non-peroxide dye solvents can assist in the removal of metallic and coating dyes from the hair. Follow the manufacturer's directions and re-test to ensure the coating is removed. The most effective guarantee of future successful services is to remove the colored hair by cutting.

SPECIAL CONSIDERATIONS FOR COLORING BLACK HAIR

As outlined in chapter 11, there are differences in hair between various races. For the hair colorist, these differences must be considered because they affect the results on the hair and the success or failure of the service.

The Cuticle

The cuticle structure of Black hair is different from that of Caucasian. One school of thought is that there are more layers of cuticle in Black hair. Another school of thought asserts that the cuticle is thicker and more tightly wound within the curve of the curl. Either way, the cuticle in Black hair is more resistant than in Caucasian hair, making it less porous. Porosity is of prime concern in hair coloring because it affects the penetration of the tint.

The Cortex The unique properties of the cortex of Black hair will affect the coloring service. The diameter of the hair is determined by the cortex. In most Black hair, this diameter is small, making the hair fine. So the hair is more resistant to penetration yet more fragile once it is softened. Pigment molecules are found within the cortex. Research indicates that the pigment molecule in Black hair is larger in size and occurs less frequently than in Caucasian hair. Because of this, Black hair is affected by lightening faster and will quickly lift with tint or lightener to a red-gold or gold stage. **Because the natural pigment is Black, however, it is very difficult to go into the lighter stages without damage to the hair.**

ANILINE DERIVATIVE TINTS The aniline derivative tints are the most widely used in hair coloring. These tints remain in the hair until they are removed by chemical means or until the hair grows out. The coloring penetrates through the cuticle into the cortex. It then binds into a complex molecule that is permanent.

An aniline derivative tint contains, as its essential ingredient, **paraphenylene-diamine** *(pah-rah-**FEN**-i-leen-**DEYE**-oh-meyen)*, or a related chemical compound. With this type of preparation, it is possible to duplicate the various shades of human hair without a loss of condition or sheen. These tints may be applied successfully over chemically processed hair.

Aniline derivative tints are sold in bottles or tubes. The stock of tints should be kept fresh, because they deteriorate on standing. Aniline derivative tints must be mixed with hydrogen peroxide to achieve lift and deposit. The peroxide causes a chemical reaction known as oxidation. This reaction begins as soon as the two compounds are mixed together, so the mixed tint must always be applied **immediately.**

Allergy to Aniline Derivatives Allergy to aniline derivative tints is an unpredictable condition. Some clients might be sensitive and others might suddenly develop a sensitivity after years of use. To identify such individuals, the U.S. Federal Food, Drug and Cosmetic Act prescribes that a **patch or predisposition test** be given 24 hours prior to application of an aniline derivative tint or toner.

> *Caution:* Aniline derivative tints must never be used on the eyelashes or eyebrows. To do so can cause blindness.

Patch Test The patch test or predisposition test must be given 24 hours before each tinting or toner treatment. The tint used for the skin test must be of the same formula as that used for the hair coloring service.

Procedure for Patch Test
1. Select the test area, either behind the ear or in the inner fold of the elbow.
2. Cleanse an area about the size of a quarter (Figure 12-4).
3. Dry the area.

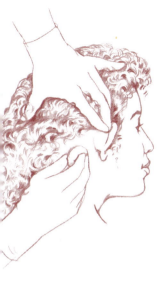

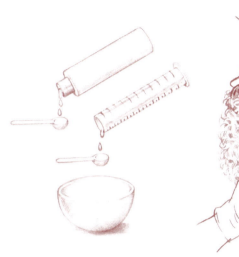

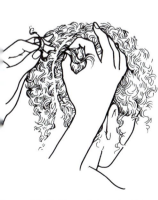

Figure 12-4. Clean patch test area.

Figure 12-5. Mix tint and peroxide.

Figure 12-6. Apply tint mixture.

4. Prepare a small amount of the test solution according to the manufacturer's directions (Figure 12-5).

5. Apply the solution to the test area with a cotton swab (Figure 12-6).

6. Leave the area undisturbed for 24 hours.

7. Examine the test area.

8. Note the results on the client's record card.

A negative skin test will show no signs of inflammation, and an aniline tint may be safely applied. A positive skin test is recognized by the presence of redness, swelling, burning, itching, and blisters. A client with such symptoms is allergic and under no circumstances should the person receive an aniline derivative tint. Application of an aniline derivative tint in this instance could result in a serious reaction for the client and a malpractice suit for the hair colorist.

Examining Scalp and Hair

Carefully examine the scalp and hair to determine if it is safe to use a hair coloring product and whether any special hair problems exist (Figure 12-7). The results of such an examination may indicate the need for any of the following:

1. Reconditioning treatment

2. Color removal

3. Removal of metallic coloring

4. Postponement of service due to breakage, and the like

5. Scalp treatment

An aniline derivative tint should not be used if the following conditions are noted:

1. Positive skin test

2. Scalp irritations or eruptions

3. Contagious scalp or hair disorders

4. Presence of metallic or compound dyes

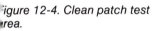

Figure 12-7. Examining scalp and hair.

The following are things to perform and consider before beginning any hair coloring process.

Consultation

Consultation is one of the most important steps in a hair coloring service. The finest formulation combined with the most talented application will still result in color failure if it is not what the client wants.

Always record the consultation on the client's record card. Perform the consultation in a well-lit room, preferably with natural lighting. If this is not possible, arrange lighting so that there is incandescent light in front of the client (around the mirror) and fluorescent light behind the colorist (ceiling fixtures). Full color fluorescent lights are also available.

When talking with the client, consider what colors will suit the skin tones and how those tones may be changing with maturity. Also consider the personality, and make sure that the color desired will not clash. Pay close attention to the described life-style so you do not select a coloring procedure that requires a great deal of care for a very active person or a color that is impractical for a client's way of life. For example, a red-gold would be the wrong choice for someone who swims regularly because chlorine can give blondish hair a green tinge. An iridescent eggplant might be the wrong choice for someone who works in a conservative law firm. Check that clients are willing to use a good quality shampoo at home that will not strip color and conditioners to maintain the condition of the hair.

The following chart will help you in your selection. Remember that each person is unique, however, and consult with your instructor.

FACTORS TO CONSIDER WHEN CHOOSING HAIR COLOR

Skin Tone Range	Eye Color	Hair Colors
Light golden brown, cafe au lait, tawny, coppery, deep golden brown, golden red brown	Hazel, green topaz, amber, cinnamon, coffee bean	Red-gold, golden brown, honey brown, chestnut, copper, auburn, mahogany, warm tones of gray, warm tones of white
Gray brown, dark brown, ebony	Gray green, deep green, brown, black	Plum, ash, ash brown, burgundy highlights, dark brown, black, slate, salt and pepper, pure white

Tint colors are usually divided into four groups:

1. Shades with no red are classified as ash (drab).
2. Shades with yellow are in the gold series. The gold series can also have warm shades that contain red.
3. Shades with red are the very warm or red series.
4. Shades with blue are classified as the cool series.

Many manufacturers include this information in their numbering system.

Basic Rules of Color Selection

1. Make sure the client's hair is clean and dry.
2. Look through the hair. To see depth as well as highlights, raise the hair by pushing it up with the hands against the scalp.
3. Analyze the depth present in the hair. Does the client want to go lighter or darker?
4. Analyze the depth of the desired color. Add or subtract from the natural color to determine the level of color necessary.
5. What are the natural highlights? What highlights does the client want? Select the color within the level that will supply those highlights or determine what primary additive should be used.
6. Know the properties of the product you are using. Consult the manufacturer's information on each color when applied to light, medium, dark hair, and so on.
7. Analyze the condition of the hair, especially its porosity. Does the hair need to be conditioned prior to the service so the color will be true and not fade?

Strand Test to Confirm Color Selection

Before applying any tint, perform a strand test to confirm your selection. You will learn the following information:

1. Whether the proper color selection was made
2. Timing to achieve desired results
3. If further pre-conditioning treatments are needed
4. If it is necessary to apply a filler

Strand Test Procedure

1. Mix 1/2 tsp of color with peroxide according to the manufacturer's directions.
2. Apply mixture to a 1/2-inch section, usually in the crown area of the head. It is important that the hair has received all pre-treatments necessary according to your analysis before the strand test is given, so that the results will be true.
3. Process with or without heat, keeping careful records of the time on the client's record card.
4. Rinse the strand, towel dry, and examine the results. Adjust the formula, timing, or preconditioning necessary and proceed with tinting on the entire head.
5. If the results are unsatisfactory, strand test again.

Following a Working Plan in Tinting

For successful hair coloring services, the technician must follow a definite procedure. A system makes for the greatest efficiency and the most satisfactory results. Without such a plan, the work takes longer, results will be uneven, and mistakes will be made.

A working plan includes the materials and supplies needed for tinting and a thorough knowledge of the product to be used. Keep a permanent record of each client's color service.

Hair Color Records

It is of the utmost importance to keep an accurate record so that any difficulties encountered in one service can be avoided in the next. Keep a complete record that contains all analysis notes, strand test, and whole head results, timing, and suggestions for the next service (Figure 12-8).

HAIR COLOR RECORD

Name.......................................Tel. ....

Address....................................City....................

Patch Test: Negative ☐   Positive ☐   Date ....

DESCRIPTION OF HAIR

Form	**Length**	**Texture**	**Pororosity**	
☐ straight	☐ short	☐ coarse	☐ very porous	☐ resistant
☐ wavy	☐ medium	☐ medium	☐ porous	☐ very resistant
☐ curly	☐ long	☐ fine	☐ normal	☐ perm. waved

Condition:

☐ normal   ☐ dry   ☐ oily   ☐ faded   ☐ streaked   ...... % gray

Previously lightened with .... for .... (time)
Previously tinted with   .... for .... (time)

☐ Original sample of hair enclosed   ☐ not enclosed

CORRECTIVE TREATMENTS
Color filler used .... Corrective treatments with ....

HAIR TINTING PROCESS
whole head ......   retouch ....inches (cm)   shade desired ....
Formula: color ....lightener ....

Results:

☐ good   ☐ poor   ☐ too light   ☐ too dark   ☐ streaked

Date	Operator	Price	Date	Operator	Price
....			....		
....			....		
....			....		

SPECIAL TECHNIQUES FOR COLORING BLACK HAIR

There are many techniques that produce great results on Black hair. The best way to achieve success is to consider the differences in the hair and alter your basic approach. If you want to deposit color, for example, plan the coloring service for the same day you relax the hair. First relax the hair as desired, then neutralize it with a deep conditioner. Rinse, then mix the conditioner with the tint for the second application. For longer staying power you can apply heat to the hair while processing. Make sure you use protective cream and avoid getting color on the scalp, which will be more sensitive after relaxing.

> **Note:** Analyze the scalp and hair completely before attempting this technique and perform any necessary patch tests. Follow all safety precautions.

Alternate Technique

Finish the relaxer completely, then apply tint that has been mixed with 5- to 10-volume peroxide. Both of these techniques can be very effective using the natural color as a base. An eggplant result, for example, can be achieved on very dark brown hair by staining with a dark auburn.

Lightening Techniques for Black Hair

When lightening Black hair, most colorists prefer to use a higher volume of peroxide, 25 to 30 volume. When used with medium- to high-level tints, lightening and brightening effects can be achieved without brassiness. A mid-level ash blonde, for example, will produce light auburn results when applied to medium brown hair.

Finishing Touches in the Coloring Procedure for Black Clients

For lasting results, any hair coloring procedure should be completed by acidifying the hair. This is also true when servicing Black clients, again with slight differences. Black hair does need to be returned to an acid pH, but without tightening the curl pattern. This is especially true for color clients who have a soft curl perm. The best result is obtained by using a manufacturer's normalizing or finishing rinse.

Always use an instant conditioner after shampooing the hair, and make sure the client buys retail products for home care.

TEMPORARY COLORS

A temporary color coats the cuticle of the hair with a film of color pigment. Since the color remains on the cuticle and does not penetrate into the cortex, it lasts only from shampoo to shampoo. Excessive porosity can allow temporary colors to penetrate, however, making it last much longer. Temporary colors usually contain certified colors that have been approved by the FDA for use in cosmetics.

Temporary colors can be used for the following advantages:

1. Bring out highlights in the hair.
2. Temporarily restore faded hair to its natural color.
3. Neutralize the yellowish tinge in white or gray hair.
4. Tone down over-lightened hair.
5. Temporarily add color to the hair without changing the structure of the hair.
6. Perform hair coloring without a skin test.

Temporary hair colorings also have several disadvantages:

1. Color is of short duration; must be applied after every shampo
2. Coating is thin and might not cover hair evenly.
3. Color might rub off on the pillow, collar, and so on, and mig run with perspiration or other moisture.
4. Can only add color, cannot lift.
5. Might result in staining if the hair is porous.

However, for the clients who want to highlight the color of their hair or glamorize gray hair, a temporary color is very helpfu Temporary colors come in various shades. Those most successfull used on Black clients include: brown, black, burgundy, blue, silver and slate. They are easily applied and are valuable as an introduction to hair coloring.

Methods of Application   There are many methods of application, depending upon th product used. Your instructor will help you interpret the manufacturer' directions.

Procedure   The hair is first shampooed and towel dried. Make sure that th client is protected by the neck strip and cape because temporar coloring can easily stain skin and clothing.

1. Have the client comfortably reclined at the shampoo bowl.
2. Apply the color. Use an applicator bottle as directed by yc instructor (Figure 12-9).
3. Apply the rinse through the entire hair shaft and comb throu (Figure 12-10).
4. Blend the color with the hair color comb; apply more color necessary.
5. DO NOT rinse the hair.
6. Proceed with styling as desired.

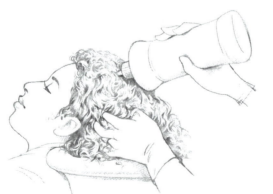

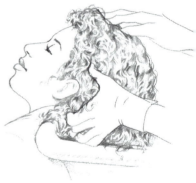

Figure 12-9. Apply temporary rinse with applicator bottle.

Figure 12-10. Distribute rinse through hair.

Cleanup   1. Discard all disposable supplies and materials.
2. Close all containers, wipe them off, and store in their proper plac
3. Clean and sanitize the implements.
4. Organize and sanitize the work area.
5. Wash and sanitize the hands.
6. File the record card.

Alternate Methods   Temporary colors are also available in the form of gels, mousses, foams, and sprays. To apply, return the client to your work area and apply color as the manufacturer directs.

SEMI-PERMANENT COLOR   Semi-permanent color offers a form of hair coloring suitable for the client who is reluctant to have a color change. The semi-permanent color is formulated to fill the gap between temporary and permanent coloring techniques.

Semi-permanent color is very often excellent for the mid-career client who thinks that his or her hair is dull, drab, or showing gray but is not ready to begin permanent hair coloring. Semi-permanent color can add highlights, blend gray, and deepen color tones without altering the natural color, since there is no lightening action on the hair.

Semi-permanent color is often chosen by younger clients as fashion fads or trends change. Semi-permanent color can deposit dramatic color or even be used for special effect streaks in bright colors. The color will naturally fade without a regrowth, so the client can change the fad color at any time or discontinue the effect.

Semi-permanent color is available in a wide range of shades. It can be purchased as a gel, cream, liquid or mousse. Results depend on the original color of the hair, the porosity, processing time, and technique.

Semi-permanent hair colors are formulated to last for four to six shampoos. No peroxide is required. The color molecules penetrate the cuticle somewhat so that the color gradually fades with each shampoo. No retouching is required. If the hair is extremely porous or if heat is used with some types of semi-permanent colors, the results can be more permanent.

Advantages of Semi-permanent Color

1. The color is self-penetrating.
2. The color is applied the same way each time.
3. Retouching is not necessary, unless the hair is extremely porous.
4. Color does not rub off on the pillow.
5. Hair will be gradually returned to its natural color after four to six shampoos.

Semi-permanent tints containing aniline derivatives require a patch test. Follow the manufacturer's instructions carefully.

Types of Semi-permanent Tints

1. Tints that cover gray completely but do not affect the remaining pigmented hair
2. Tints that make gray hair more beautiful without changing the natural pigment
3. Tints that add color and highlights to hair that is not gray
4. Translucent tints that add gloss, highlights, and sometimes special effects to the hair. These colors vary in their effect according to porosity, heat application, and timing. Consult your instructor and the product information for assistance with these products.
5. Regular tints that are mixed with conditioning agents rather than peroxide. These "stains" may be used as semi-permanent colors or toners.

Preliminary Steps

1. Give a preliminary patch test if required. Proceed only if the test is negative.
2. Thoroughly analyze the hair and scalp. Record the results on the client record card.
3. Assemble all the necessary supplies.
4. Prepare the client. Protect the clothing with a towel and tint cape. Have the client remove jewelry and put it safely away.
5. Apply protective cream around the hairline and over the ears.
6. Put on protective gloves.
7. Perform a strand test.
8. Record the results on the client's card.

Procedure

1. Give a mild shampoo, if required.
2. Towel dry the hair.
3. Put on protective gloves.
4. Apply tint to the entire hair shaft, starting near the scalp and gently working the color through the ends. Apply with a bottle or brush according to the consistency of the color selected and your instructor's directions (Figures 12-11 and 12-12).
5. Pile the hair loosely on top of the head.
6. Follow the manufacturer's directions as to whether to use a plastic cap, heat, and so on (Figure 12-13).
7. Process according to the strand test results.
8. When the color has developed, wet the hair with tepid water and lather.

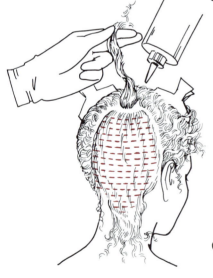

Figure 12-11. Apply semi-permanent color.

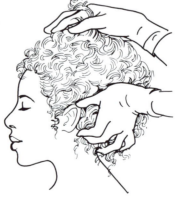

Figure 12-12. Gently work color through hair.

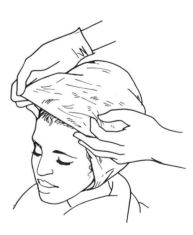

Figure 12-13. Use plastic covering if required.

9. Rinse with warm water until the water runs clear (Figure 12-14).

10. Give a finishing rinse to close the cuticle and set the color (Figure 12-15).

11. Rinse and towel blot hair. Style as desired.

12. Complete the record card and file.

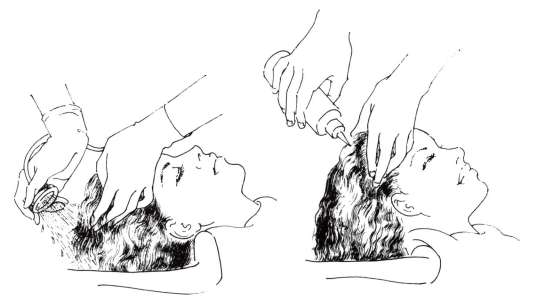

Figure 12-14. Rinse with warm water until water runs clear.

Figure 12-15. Give finishing rinse.

Cleanup

1. Discard all disposable supplies and materials.

2. Close all containers, wipe them off, and store safely.

3. Clean and sanitize the implements.

4. Clean and sanitize the tint cape.

5. Sanitize the work area.

6. Wash and sanitize the hands.

7. Complete the record card and file.

PERMANENT HAIR COLOR

Practically all permanent hair coloring is done with oxidizing penetrating tints that contain aniline derivatives. These tints penetrate the cuticle of the hair and enter the cortical layer. Here, they are oxidized by the peroxide added into color pigments. These pigments are distributed throughout the hair shaft much like natural pigment.

Penetrating tints are also referred to as:

1. Single-process or single-application tints.

2. Double-process or double-application tints.

Single-process tints lighten and/or deposit color in a single application. Basic tints are formulated to perform both lift and deposit functions, but the technician can use them in such a way that either lift only or deposit only is achieved. Deposit-only tints are also available; they are formulated with no lift capacity.

Single-process tints can be purchased in a variety of forms. Liquid tints were the first available and are still used today for many basic color applications. Cream formulas add conditioning agents for slightly damaged hair. Creams also give a thicker consistency so the color does not run onto the client's skin. Gels and very thick creams that come in tubes can also be purchased. Some colorists prefer them for gray hair or special effects. Your instructor can help you decide which is best for your client.

Double-process tints perform only one activity at a time. They require two separate and distinct applications to the hair:

1. The application of a softener or lightener.
2. The application of a tint or toner.

As a safety precaution, a skin or patch test must be given before tinting the hair. The colorist should wear protective gloves, and the client should be draped to protect clothing.

Single-Process Tints

Single-process tints represent a simplified method of hair coloring. Both lift and deposit can occur at one time to achieve the desired color. Pre-lightening or pre-softening is not required.

Single-process tints usually contain a lightening agent, shampoo, aniline derivative tint and an alkalizing agent to activate the peroxide that is added. Most color is formulated to be used with 20 volume peroxide. When working with Black hair you might have to use 2 to 30 percent volume, especially if you want to lighten the hair. Be guided by your instructor because color results are altered when volumes other than those specified by the manufacturer are used.

The following are advantages of single-process tints:

1. Produce shades from deep black to blonde
2. Color the hair lighter or darker than the client's original shade
3. Blend white or gray hair to a natural hair shade
4. Correct streaks, off-shades, discolorations, and faded ends
5. Can be purchased in cream, liquid and gel form

Single-Process Tint Lightening Procedure for Virgin Hair

Virgin hair is hair that has had no chemical services, no pressing damage, and has not been damaged by natural factors such as wind, sun, and so on.

The procedure that follows is a basic color procedure (Figures 12-16 through 12-18). Your instructor might have another technique that is just as appropriate for the particular color used.

Implements and Materials

Towels	Mild shampoo
Tint cape	Selected tint
Protective gloves	Hydrogen peroxide
Comb	Color chart
Record card	Finishing rinse
Talcum powder	Protective cream
Applicator (brush, bottle, or bowl)	Cotton
Timer	

Preliminary Steps

1. Give a patch test 24 hours before the service. Proceed only if the test is negative.
2. Thoroughly analyze the scalp and hair. Perform any necessary preconditioning treatments and record the results on the client's record card.
3. Assemble all necessary supplies.
4. Prepare the client. Protect the clothing with a towel and tint cape. Have the client remove all jewelry and put it safely away.
5. Apply protective cream around the hairline and over the ears.
6. Put on protective gloves.
7. Perform a strand test.
8. Record the results on a record card.

Helpful Suggestions

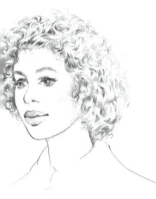

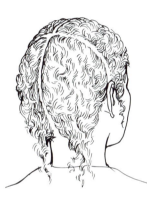

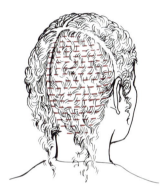

Figure 12-16a Client draped

Figure 12-16. Section hair into four parts.

Figure 12-16c Subdivide sections into one-quarter- inch sections.

Procedure

1. Section the hair into four quarters.
2. Prepare the tint formula.
3. Begin in the section where the color change will be the greatest.
4. Part off a 1/4-inch subsection with the applicator.
5. Lift a subsection and apply the tint to the hair 1 inch from the scalp up to but not through the ends (usually 1 inch). The hair at the scalp will process faster due to body heat and incomplete keratinization. For this reason the tint is applied in the scalp area after the center shaft. Color will penetrate and process faster on the ends due to porosity. Your strand test will determine application procedure and timing for even color development.
6. Process the tint according to the strand results.
7. Apply the tint mixture to the hair near the scalp, being careful to avoid contact with the scalp.
8. Apply the tint to the hair ends.
9. Process according to the strand test results and confirm development by removing the color from the strand.
10. Lightly rinse with lukewarm water. Massage color to lather and rinse thoroughly.

11. Remove stains around the hairline with the remaining tint mixtu[re], shampoo, or stain remover. Use cotton to gently remove stain[s].
12. Shampoo the hair thoroughly with a mild (acid-balanced) shampo[o].
13. Apply an acid or a finishing rinse to close the cuticle, resto[re] pH, and prevent fading.
14. Style the hair.
15. Complete the record card and file.

Bottle Application

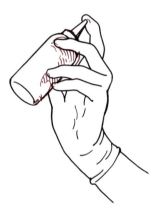

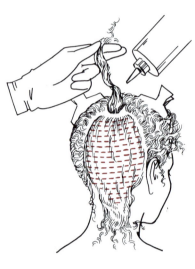

Figure 12-17a. Prepare the mixture; shake the bottle gently.

Figure 12-17b. Apply tint to a one-quarter-inch strand.

Brush Application

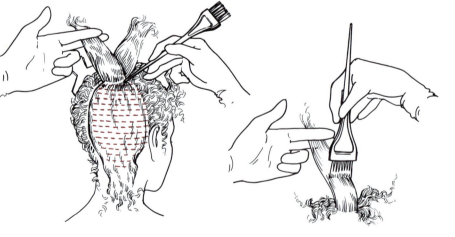

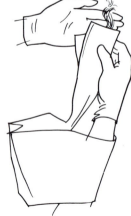

Figure 12-18a. Part a one-quarter-inch section with a tint brush.

Figure 12-18b. Apply tint to each subsection top and bottom.

Figure 12-18c. Strand testing for color development.

Cleanup
1. Discard all disposable supplies and materials.
2. Close all containers tightly, wipe them off, and put them in their proper places.
3. Clean and sanitize the implements.
4. Sanitize the tint cape.
5. Sanitize the work area.
6. Wash and sanitize the hands.

Tinting to a Darker Shade

When tinting close to or darker than the natural hair color, follow the same preparation and procedure as for a lighter shade, with the following exceptions:
1. Select the appropriate color.
2. Apply tint from the hair closest to the scalp to the ends.
3. Check for development according to the strand test and complete in the usual manner.

SINGLE-PROCESS TINT RETOUCH

As the hair grows, you will need to do a *retouch* so the hair is attractive and not two-toned. After you assemble the materials and implements as if for a virgin tint, follow the procedure below.

Preliminary Steps
1. Give a patch test 24 hours before the service. Proceed only if the test is negative.
2. Assemble all necessary supplies.
3. Prepare the client. Protect the clothing with a towel and tint cape. Have the client remove all jewelry and put it safely away.
4. Remove the client's record card. Consult with the client to see if she or he liked the original color. Carefully analyze the hair and condition previously tinted hair as needed.
5. Apply protective cream around the hairline and over the ears.
6. Perform a strand test.
7. Record all results on a record card.

Procedure
1. Section the hair into four quarters.
2. Prepare the tint formula.
3. Begin in the section where color change will be greatest.
4. Part off a 1/4-inch subsection with the applicator.
5. Apply tint to the new growth only. DO NOT OVERLAP. Overlapping of color can cause breakage and lines of demarcation (Figure 12-19).
6. Process the tint according to the strand test results.
7. Apply diluted color formula to the ends according to your analysis and strand test results. Dilute the remaining tint mixture with distilled water, shampoo, or conditioner.

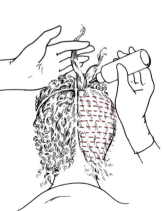

Figure 12-19. Retouching new growth.

8. Lightly rinse with lukewarm water. Massage color to lather ar rinse thoroughly.

9. Remove any stains around the hairline with the remaining ti mixture, shampoo or stain remover. Use cotton to gently remo the stains.

10. Shampoo the hair thoroughly with a mild (acid balanced) shampc

11. Apply an acid or a finishing rinse to close the cuticle, resto the pH, and prevent fading.

12. Complete the record card and file.

HIGHLIGHTING SHAMPOO COLORS

Highlighting shampoo tints are prepared by combining anilin derivative tints, hydrogen peroxide, and shampoo. They are use when a very slight change in hair shade is desired or when th client's hair processes very rapidly. These tints highlight the hair natural color in a single application. A patch test is required.

Highlighting shampoos are a mixture of shampoo and hydroge peroxide. The natural color is slightly lightened. No patch test i required.

Procedure

Perform consultation and analysis as for regular color procedure If highlighting shampoo tint is to be used, a patch test must have been performed 24 hours before.

Drape the client and take him or her to the shampoo bowl. Distribute the color over clean, damp hair. Gently lather and process for to 15 minutes (Figure 12-20).

Complete as a regular tint procedure.

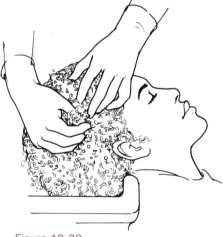

Figure 12-20
Applying highlighting shampoo color.

PRE-LIGHTENING OR PRE-SOFTENING

If the client desires a drastically lighter color, the hair should firs be pre-lightened. The pre-lightener is applied in the same manne as that for a regular hair lightening treatment.

After the pre-lightening has reached the desired stage, the hai is lightly shampooed, acidified, and towel dried. The color is ther applied in the usual manner, after a strand test has been made

Pre-softening is very effective on Black hair, which tends to be resistant. Resistant hair must be pre-softened in order for it to readily absorb tint.

Apply the softener from the scalp to the hair ends as in a regular lightening process and process a few minutes. Little color change will take place, but the cuticle is opened so that the hair is more receptive to color. Do not rinse softener from hair. Towel blot and apply color as the manufacturer directs.

TIPS AND SAFETY PRECAUTIONS FOR COLORING BLACK HAIR

1. Use extreme care when lightening Black hair.
2. Permanently colored or lightened Black hair will always have warmth in it, no matter what shade of tint is used.
3. The darker or finer your client's hair, the more red or gold will be visible after coloring or lightening.
4. Avoid lightening beyond a red-gold stage because it will almost always cause damage to the Black client's hair.
5. If the client's hair is damaged, be sure to recondition his or her hair before giving a coloring service.
6. Remember to use between 25 to 30 percent volume peroxide when coloring your client's hair.
7. Do not lighten Black hair that has been chemically treated with perms or relaxers.

GENERAL SAFETY PRECAUTIONS FOR COLORING AND LIGHTENING

1. Give a patch test 24 hours prior to any application of aniline derivatives.
2. Apply tint only if the patch test is negative.
3. Do not apply tint if abrasions are present.
4. Do not apply tint if metallic or compound dye is present.
5. Do not brush hair prior to coloring.
6. Always read and follow the manufacturer's directions.
7. Use sanitized applicator bottles, brushes, combs, and towels.
8. Protect the client's clothing by proper draping.
9. Take a strand test for color, breakage, and/or discoloration.
10. Use an applicator bottle or bowl (glass or plastic) for mixing the tint.
11. Do not mix the tint before you are ready to use it; discard leftover tint.
12. Wear gloves to protect your hands.
13. Do not permit the color to come in contact with the client's eyes.
14. Do not overlap during a tint retouch.
15. Do not use water that is too hot; use lukewarm water for removing color.
16. Use a mild shampoo. If an alkaline or harsh shampoo is used it will strip the color.
17. Always wash your hands before and after serving a client.

1. What are five reasons for coloring or lightening hair?
2. What are the four classifications of hair coloring?
3. How do pigment molecules in Black hair differ from pigmen molecules in Caucasian hair?
4. What is the procedure for an aniline derivative tint patch test
5. What are the basic rules of color selection?
6. Which volume of peroxide do most colorists prefer to use o Black hair?
7. What are the advantages and disadvantages of temporary ha colorings?
8. What is the procedure for semi-permanent hair coloring?
9. How do you apply a single-process tint?
10. What is the procedure for a single-process tint retouch?
11. How are lightening shampoo tints prepared?
12. What does pre-softening do to the hair?
13. What are five tips and safety precautions for coloring Black hair
14. What are twelve general safety precautions for coloring an lightening?

Chapter 13 Hair Lightening and Other Color Techniques

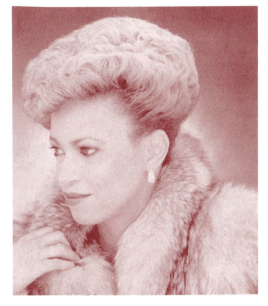

LEARNING OBJECTIVES   After you have mastered this chapter, you will be able to:

1. List the four stages of lightening appropriate for the Black client.
2. Explain what happens to the brown pigment in Black hair once lightener is applied.
3. Give the three types of hair lightener.
4. Explain the three uses of hydrogen peroxide and how it is activated.
5. Give the procedure for lightening virgin hair.
6. Tell where lightener is applied during a retouch.
7. List twelve lightener safety precautions.
8. List seven conditions that show hair is damaged.
9. Give the advantage of color fillers.
10. Explain the procedure for tint removal.
11. Give the procedure for a tint back.
12. Define allergy, developer, lift, overlapping, oxidation, prelightening, and resistant hair.

INTRODUCTION   Hair lightening involves the partial or total diffusion of the natural pigment of artificial color in the hair. Hair lightening removes pigment from the hair. Changing styles will determine if the lightening is over the whole head, in one area, or a special effect. Remember that lightening your Black client's hair beyond the red-gold stage will almost always cause damage to hair. Try to discourage clients who are considering a tone or shade that requires lightening beyond this stage. If your analysis of skin tone and hair condition permits you to lighten further, discourage your client from using any chemical relaxers.

Lighteners may be used for the following purposes:

1. As a color treatment, to lighten hair to the final shade desire
2. As a preliminary treatment, to prepare hair for the application
   a tint (double-process application)
   a. Toner—A lightener is always necessary before applyir
      delicate toner shades. For a toner to have visible results, Blac
      hair would have to be lightened past the red-gold stag
      Because taking the hair past that stage is almost alway
      inadvisable when working on Black hair, toners are seldo
      necessary when servicing Black clients.
   b. Tint—If the client desires a shade much lighter than the natur
      shade, a lightener can be used to remove some color befo
      the tint is applied.

Hair lighteners, depending upon the manufacturer's directions, ar
used on Black clients to do the following:

1. Lighten hair to a particular shade
2. Brighten and lighten the existing shade
3. Lighten only certain parts of the hair
4. Lighten hair that has already been tinted
5. Remove undesirable casts and off-shades
6. Correct dark streaks or spots in lightened or tinted hair

Effects of Lighteners

A lightening product is used to lift hair to a desired shade. The
hair pigment goes through different changing stages of color as I
lightens. The amount of change depends on the pigmentation c
the hair and the length of time the lightening agent is processed
For example: A natural head of black hair will go from black to brown
to red, to red-gold, to gold, to yellow, and finally to pale yellow (almos
white). The four stages of lightening appropriate for the Black clien
are illustrated (Figures 13-1a through 13-1d) below.

a. Black

b. Brown

c. Red

d. Red-gold

The hair also becomes more porous during the lightening treatment, a condition that facilitates the penetration of a tint (Figure 13-2).

Figure 13-2 **Action of hair lighteners.**

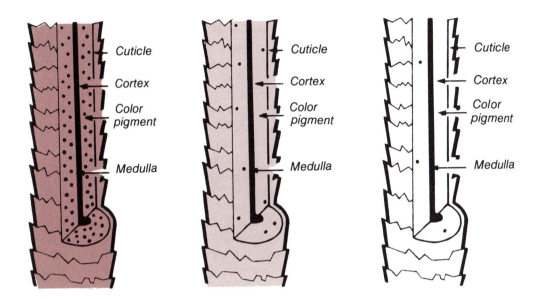

Cuticle

Cortex

Color pigment

Medulla

Cuticle

Cortex

Color pigment

Medulla

Cuticle

Cortex

Color pigment

Medulla

Problems in Hair Lightening

The natural color of hair is determined by its pigment content. Natural hair coloring has either brown or yellow and red pigments or a mixture.

Never promise a Black client that dark hair can be lightened to a pale blonde shade.

Brown pigment changes to a lighter shade a few minutes after application of the lightener. In Black hair, this pigment is larger and will lighten to the red-gold stage very rapidly once lightener has penetrated the cortex.

Red pigment is diffused in the cortex. It must be shattered to obtain pale tones, a procedure that might damage your client's hair.

Yellow pigment presents the least problems, but it can lift unevenly, causing streaks.

It is important to select the right lightener for good results. Always make a strand test to gauge results. Consult the manufacturer's information and follow that and your instructor's directions.

TYPES OF LIGHTENERS

Lighteners are available in oil, cream, and powder forms.

The cosmetologist must know how each type works as well as when to use a particular kind.

Oil Lighteners

Oil lighteners are usually mixtures of hydrogen peroxide and sulfonated oil. They are usually slow acting and designed to be used for lightening the entire head. Caution should be used because these lighteners can run and drip.

Cream and Gel Lighteners

Cream and gel lighteners are the most popular types. They are easily applied and will not run, drip, or dry out easily. They are easy to control and contain conditioning agents, sometimes bluing, and thickener. The benefits of cream lighteners are as follows:

1. Conditioning agents give some protection to the hair and scalp
2. Bluing agents help drab red and gold tones.
3. Thickeners give more control during application.
4. Cream does not swell, so it helps prevent overlapping during retouch.

Powder Lighteners

Powder lighteners, also called quick lighteners, contain oxygen releasing boosters for quicker and stronger action. Paste lighteners dry out more quickly, but they do not run or drip. Most powder lighteners are too harsh to use on the hair closest to the scalp so they are used for special effects lightening. Most powder lighteners swell as processing continues and should not be used for retouch services. Powder lighteners are recommended for resistant hair.

HYDROGEN PEROXIDE

The lightening agent for removing pigment from the hair shaft is hydrogen peroxide (H_2O_2), which is activated by the addition of an alkali. The active ingredient of hydrogen peroxide is oxygen gas. The oxygen gas surrounds the hair pigment. It then reflects a lighter color to the eye. As the lightener processes longer or when boosters or high-volume peroxide are used, the pigment molecule is shattered reflecting blonde tones.

Volume refers to the capacity of the hydrogen peroxide. One liter of 20-volume peroxide, for example, is capable of releasing 20 liters of free oxygen gas, ten liters of oxygen, and so on. Higher volumes are used for more lift, lower volumes for more deposit. Most manufacturer's colors will produce the chart results on white hair when mixed with 20-volume peroxide. As mentioned before, when coloring Black hair, 25- to 30-volume peroxide gives better results. The technician must always consider the natural pigment present to determine the results.

When properly used, hydrogen peroxide can lighten and soften hair without damage. Use of higher volume peroxide can damage the cuticle, so after treatment conditioning is necessary. Repeated use of lighteners can make hair dry and damaged, so each service should include reconditioning.

Hydrogen peroxide is available in liquid, cream, gel, and tablet form. Peroxide should be kept in a cool, dry place.

Do not permit peroxide to come in contact with metal. When liquid peroxide is kept too long, exposed to air, stored in a warm place or contaminated, its strength weakens.

Uses of Hydrogen Peroxide

As a softener, peroxide can lift the cuticle imbrications to make hair more receptive to the penetration of a tint.

As an oxidizer, a hydrogen peroxide solution is used in permanent aniline tints. The oxygen links the color molecules together to tint the hair.

LIGHTENING VIRGIN HAIR

A preliminary strand test is necessary when lightening to determine the processing time, the condition of the hair after lightening, and the end results. Carefully record all data on the client's record card.

Preliminary Test Results

1. If the test shows the hair is not light enough:
   a) Increase the strength of the mixture and/or
   b) Increase the processing time
2. If the hair strand is too light:
   a) Decrease the strength of the mixture and/or
   b) Decrease the processing time
3. Watch the strand carefully for reaction to lightening mixture, discoloration, and breakage.
4. If color and condition are good, proceed with lightening.

Procedure

The following general instructions might be changed by your instructor for particular lightening effects or products.

1. Prepare the client. Protect the client's clothing with a towel and tint cape.
2. Analyze the scalp and hair and record on the client's card. Do not perform the service if the client has abrasions or inflammation of the scalp. Do not brush the hair.
3. Section the hair into four equal parts (Figure 13-3).
4. Apply protective cream around the hairline and over the ears.
5. Put on protective gloves.
6. Prepare lightening formula and use immediately to prevent deterioration.
7. Apply the lightener. Begin the application where the hair seems resistant, usually at the back of the head. Use 1/8-inch partings to apply the lightener. Start about 1/2 to 1 inch from the scalp and extend the lightener to the point where the hair shafts show signs of damage (the ends). Apply lightener to the top and underside of the subsection in a quick, rhythmic movement (Figures 13-4 and 13-5).

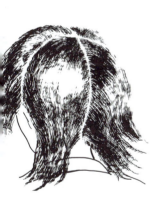

Figure 13-3. Section hair into four equal parts.

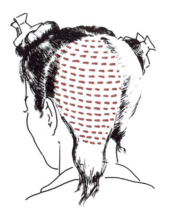

Figure 13-4. Applying lightener to the underside of the strand.

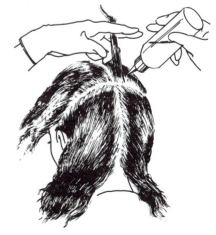

Figure 13-5. Applying lightener to the scalp area.

153

8. Continue to apply lightener until all of the center shaft area saturated. Double-check the application, adding more lightener if necessary. Do not comb the lightener through the hair. Keep the lightener moist during development by misting hair lightly with a spray bottle or reapplying lightener as the mixture dries.

9. Test for lightening action. Make the first check about 15 minutes before the time indicated by the preliminary strand test. Remove the mixture from the strand with a damp towel. Towel dry and examine. If the strand is not light enough, reapply the mixture and continue to test frequently until the desired level is reached.

10. Apply the lightener to the hair near the scalp. If necessary, prepare fresh lightener. Use 1/8-inch partings and avoid overlapping previously lightened hair. When the scalp area is processed sufficiently, apply the remaining mixture to the hair ends. Pile the hair loosely on the head and cover with a plastic cap if directed. Strand test until the entire hair shaft has reached the desired stage.

11. Remove the lightener. Rinse thoroughly with cool water. Shampoo gently with an acid-balanced shampoo. Be certain to shampoo with your hands under the hair to avoid tangling.

12. Neutralize the alkalinity of the hair with an acid or a normalizing rinse.

13. Towel dry hair or completely dry under a cool dryer if the manufacturer requires it.

14. Examine the scalp for abrasions. Analyze the condition of the hair. Recondition if necessary.

15. Complete the record card file.

16. Clean up in the usual manner.

LIGHTENER RETOUCH

As the hair grows, dark regrowth will be very obvious. A lightener retouch corrects this problem and matches the regrowth to the rest of the lightened hair.

During the retouch, the lightener is applied to the new growth only with the following exceptions:

1. Another color is desired.

2. A lighter shade is desired.

3. Color has become dull from repeated applications.

In each case, lighten the regrowth first. Then bring the remaining lightener mixture gently through the hair shaft. Process 1 to 5 minutes until the problem is corrected.

Retouch Procedure

The client record card is a guide for lightener formula, timing, and the like. A cream lightener is generally used for a lightener retouch because its consistency helps prevent overlapping of previously lightened hair and it is gentler on the scalp.

This procedure for a lightener retouch is the same as that for lightening a virgin head of hair, except that the mixture is applied only to the new growth of hair (Figures 13-6 through 13-8).

Care should be taken not to overlap the lightener onto previously lightened hair. Overlapping can cause severe breakage and lines of demarcation.

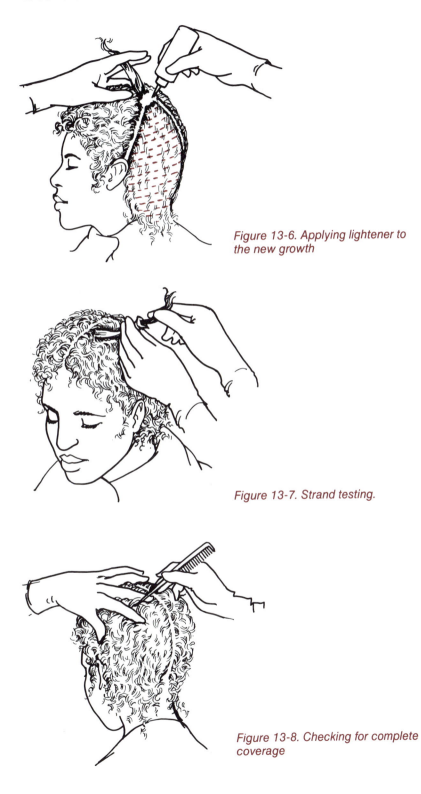

Figure 13-6. Applying lightener to the new growth

Figure 13-7. Strand testing.

Figure 13-8. Checking for complete coverage

1. Read the manufacturer's directions before preparing lightener.
2. Always wash your hands before and after servicing a client.
3. Drape a client properly to protect clothing. Use only sanitize applicators and towels.
4. Examine the scalp carefully. Do not apply lightener if irritatic or abrasions are present.
5. Do not brush the hair. If shampoo is required, avoid irritating th scalp.
6. Analyze the condition of the hair and give any necessary r conditioning treatments.
7. Wear protective gloves.
8. Strand test before the lightener retouch.
9. Cream lightener should be the thickness of whipped cream avoid dripping, running, or overlapping.
10. Always use lightener immediately after mixing. Discard leftov lightener.
11. Apply lightener to the resistant areas first. Use 1/8-inch parting to ensure accurate coverage.
12. Apply rapidly and neatly for even lightening.
13. Take frequent strand tests until the desired stage is reached.
14. Check the skin and scalp after application and gently remov any lightener with a cool, damp towel.
15. If the towel around the client's neck becomes saturated, remov and replace to avoid skin irritation.
16. Cool water and mild shampoo should be used to remove th lightener.
17. Cap all bottles to avoid contamination.
18. Complete a record card and file.

Spot Lightening

Uneven lightening, streaking, or dark spots are usually due to careless lightener application. To correct streaked hair, do the following:

1. Prepare the lightening formula.
2. Apply the mixture only to the darker areas.
3. Allow the mixture to remain on the hair until all streaks are remove
4. Shampoo the lightener from the hair.

**SPECIAL PROBLEMS IN
HAIR COLORING**

Each coloring service is unique. The colorist must carefully analyze the hair and consult the client. Strand tests must be taken to ensure good results.

But even skilled colorists will occasionally have a hair coloring problem. This can be due to the service attempted or to a prio service received at home or elsewhere.

Damaged Hair   Blow-drying, pressing, harsh shampoos, chemical services, and so forth, all take their toll on the condition of the hair. Coating compounds such as hair spray, styling agents, activators, and some conditioners can prevent penetration of the color. Preventive and corrective steps that you should take include the following:

1. Incorporate reconditioning in any chemical service that you give.
2. Ensure that the client uses quality product at home by retailing.
3. Pre-condition hair if your analysis tells you it is damaged. Use a penetrating conditioner that can deposit protein, oils, moisture regulators, and so on.
4. Complete any chemical service by normalizing the pH with a finishing rinse.
5. Postpone any further chemical service until the hair is reconditioned.
6. Schedule the client for between-service conditioning.

Hair is considered damaged when it has one or more of the following conditions:

1. Over-porous
2. Brittle and dry
3. Breakage
4. No elasticity
5. Spongy, matted when wet
6. Color fades or absorbs too rapidly
7. Rough texture

Any of the above hair conditions can create trouble during tinting, lightening or any other chemical service. Therefore, damaged hair should receive reconditioning treatments prior to and after the application of chemical agents.

Reconditioning
Procedure

1. Always thoroughly analyze the hair to determine the problem. Consult with the client until you can discover the cause of the damage. Then you can correct the problem and stop it from recurring.
2. Wash the hair with a mild shampoo. Keep your hands underneath the hair and use only gentle massage techniques to avoid tangling the fragile hair.
3. Rinse very well and towel blot gently.
4. Apply the conditioner as the manufacturer requires. If it is a liquid, use a spray bottle; if it is a cream, apply with a sanitized spatula or tint brush.
5. Blend the conditioner through the hair with a wide-tooth comb.
6. Cover the hair with a plastic cap if required and follow the manufacturer's directions for applying heat and the timing.
7. Rinse well. Reexamine the hair and proceed with the coloring service only if its condition indicates the coloring will be successful.

FILLERS   Fillers are specialized preparations that are designed to equaliz porosity and deposit a base color in one application. They can b a preparation from the manufacturer or a mixture of tint and condition that your instructor will assist you in preparing.

Conditioner fillers are used to recondition damaged hair befor salon service. Conditioner fillers can be applied in a separat procedure as outlined above or applied immediately prior to col application. The conditioner and the tint are then working at the sam time.

Color fillers are recommended if the hair is damaged and ther is doubt that the color result will be an even shade.

Advantages of Color Fillers

1. Deposit color to the faded ends
2. Help hair to hold the color
3. Help the color to develop uniformly from scalp to ends
4. Prevent streaking
5. Prevent off-color results
6. Prevent dullness
7. Give more uniform, natural-looking color

How to Use Color Fillers   Color fillers may be applied directly from their containers to th damaged hair prior to tinting. Color fillers may be added to the ti and applied to damaged ends. They may also be used full strengt or diluted with distilled water.

Selection of Correct Color Filler   To obtain satisfactory results, select the color filler that will replac a missing primary. Always remember that all three primaries--red blue, and yellow--must be present for natural looking hair color. Fo example, if you have red-gold hair being tinted back to black, yo will need a blue filler so that the end result will be correct.

TINT REMOVAL   Sometimes it is necessary to remove all or part of the tint fro the hair to achieve the correct color.

Commercial products used to remove penetrating tints are know as tint or color removers. They may contain color strippers, liftin agents, and are sometimes mixed with hydrogen peroxide.

The removal of tint is always an advanced technique that require careful analysis of both the condition and color of the hai Reconditioning is often necessary after tint removal and befor corrective color is applied.

Procedure

1. Prepare the client.
2. Shampoo if required by the manufacturer.
3. Section the hair into four equal quarters.
4. Put on protective gloves.
5. Mix the preparation in a glass or plastic bowl according to t manufacturer's directions.

6. Immediately begin application where the hair is darkest (Figure 13-9).

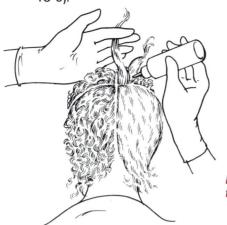

Figure 13-9. Applying mixture to the darkest area

7. Apply the mixture with a tint brush. Saturate the hair completely.
8. Strand test immediately. Test frequently as the hair processes.

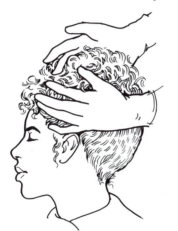

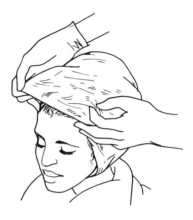

Figure 13-10. Piling hair on top of hair

Figure 13-11. Applying a plastic cap to speed processing.

9. Pile the hair loosely on top of the head and cover with a plastic cap if required (Figures 13-10 and 13-11).
10. Per the manufacturer's directions, apply heat to speed the processing.

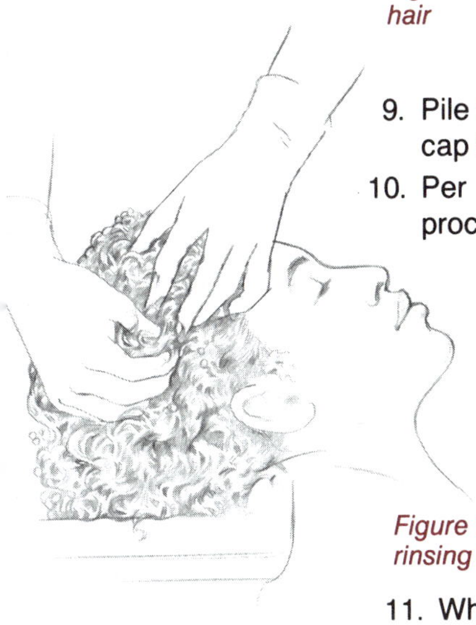

Figure 13-12. Shampooing and rinsing thoroughly with cool water

11. When the color is removed, shampoo thoroughly (Figure 13-12).

12. Rinse thoroughly to ensure all of the chemical is removed fro the hair. Any tint remover that remains in the hair will contin to process.

13. Towel dry the hair.

14. Analyze the hair strength. Condition as required.

15. Perform a strand test.

16. Proceed with the application of desired tint.

If color cannot be applied, style the hair in the usual manner Schedule reconditioning treatments until the hair can withstand tinting

Removing Coating Dyes   Dyes, such as metallic and compound, vegetable tints, and some semi-permanent tints coat the hair shaft rather than penetrate i Regular chemical services cannot be given to the client until the coating layer is removed. Commercial dye removers are sometimes successful in removing these coatings, although success cannot be guaranteed. It is often necessary to remove the coated hair by cutting before chemical services can be successful.

TINT BACK TO NATURAL COLOR   Each tint back to natural color must be handled as an individua problem. Check the hair for its natural color next to the scalp. Carefully consult with the client to see if she or he is ready for a color tha dark. You will sometimes have to compromise with a color that has the same color qualities but is lighter in value. Carefully record a observations and treatments on the client's record card.

Procedure
1. Assemble the materials.
2. Prepare the client in the usual manner.
3. Check the results of the patch test. Proceed only if results ar negative.
4. Shampoo the hair as directed and give conditioning treatment according to your analysis.
5. Perform a strand test. More than one test might be necessar
6. Section the hair into four equal quarters.
7. Apply the filler as directed by your instructor. Remember to replac the missing primary.
8. Process the filler according to the manufacturer's directions. Towe blot excess filler. Proceed directly to the tint application.
9. Resection the hair into four equal quarters.
10. Apply color formula to 1/4-inch subsections. Apply the tint a rapidly as possible to both sides of the subsection from scal to ends.
11. Check for complete coverage.
12. Test for color development immediately. Check frequently unt the desired shade is reached.
13. Remove the tint from the hair with a mild shampoo.
14. Use an acid rinse to close the cuticle and prevent fading.
15. Replace moisture with a finishing rinse.
16. Style as desired, using caution to avoid excessive heat o stretching.

17. Retail quality products that will prevent color stripping at home, and schedule the client for conditioning treatments.
18. Complete a record card and file.
19. Clean the work area in the usual manner.

DEFINITIONS PERTAINING TO HAIR COLORING

Accelerating (Processing) Machine: Equipment used to speed the processing of a tint or lightener.

Allergy: Skin sensitivity to cosmetics, tints, foods, or other substances. In hair coloring, a very small number of clients might be allergic to aniline derivative tints.

Blending: The process of making the color uniform throughout the hair.

Coating: Building up of a product on the outside of the hair.

Color Filler: A preparation containing a base color used to equalize porosity in the hair so that it will take and hold color evenly.

Conditioner: Cosmetic applied to hair to restore strength, elasticity, manageability, and sheen.

Decolorization: The removal of natural and artificial color pigment from the hair.

Developer: An oxidizing agent, such as hydrogen peroxide, that releases oxygen to activate tint molecules or to lift pigment from the hair.

Development Time: Processing time for desired color development.

Frosting, Tipping, Streaking: Techniques for partial lightening of small sections of hair on various parts of the head.

Heating Cap: Electrical cap sometimes used to hasten the coloring process.

Highlighting: A brightening effect accomplished by the application of a high lift tint or lightener to selected strands within a style.

Hydrometer (Peroxometer): Instrument used to measure the volume of hydrogen peroxide.

Lift: The potential lightening of a tint or lightener.

Line of Demarcation: Streak caused by overlapping previously tinted or lightened hair. Also a term used to indicate the end of new hair growth.

Overlapping: Condition caused in a retouch by having a tint or lightener overlap any previously treated hair. Can cause breakage or a line of demarcation.

Oxidation: Chemical reaction of released oxygen combining with another substance. This takes place when peroxide and the tinting solution are mixed and applied to the hair.

Patch or Skin Test: Procedure for determining an allergic reaction to an aniline derivative tint.

Porosity: The ability of the hair to absorb moisture due to lifted cuticle layers.

Powder Lightener: A strong, fast-acting lightener used for special effects and off-the-scalp lightening.

Pre-lightening: The process of removing color from the hair before a tint application.

Pre-softening: The application of a lightener to soften resistant hair and make it more receptive to color.

Record Card: A written record of each client's hair structur[e], condition, chemical service, and results.

Resistant Hair: Hair with a tightly packed cuticle that is slow [to] process.

Retouch: The application of color or lightener to the new grow[th] of hair.

Semi-permanent Hair Coloring: Hair coloring formulated to la[st] from four to six shampoos. It penetrates the hair shaft slight[ly] depending upon the porosity of the hair. It uses no peroxide f[or] development.

Sensitivity: Condition when the skin reacts to a chemical b[y] becoming red and irritated.

Soap Cap: A mixture of tint with shampoo, worked through th[e] hair as a shampoo.

Spot Lightening: Application of lightener only to dark areas [to] even out the color.

Spot Tinting: Application of tint to areas insufficiently colored [to] achieve even results.

Strand Test: Preliminary color application to a small subsectio[n] of hair. Predetermines mixture, development time, and results.

Stripping: Term used to indicate the removal of natural ha[ir] pigment, coating, or penetrating tint from the hair.

Tint Back: Coloring the hair back to its natural shade.

Tint Removal: The use of dye solvent, lightener, or softenin[g] treatment to remove an unsatisfactory shade of tint from the ha[ir].

Virgin Hair: Hair that has never received a chemical treatme[nt].

QUESTIONS FOR REVIEW

1. Which four stages of lightening are appropriate for the Black clie[nt]?
2. What happens to the brown pigment in Black hair, once lighte[ner] is applied?
3. What are the three types of hair lighteners?
4. How is hydrogen peroxide activated and what are its three us[es] in hair coloring?
5. What is the procedure for lightening virgin hair?
6. Where is lightener applied during a retouch?
7. What are twelve lightener safety precautions?
8. What are seven conditions that show hair is damaged?
9. What are the advantages of color fillers?
10. How is tint removed from the hair?
11. What is the procedure for a tint back?
12. What are the definitions of allergy, developer, lift, overlapp[ing] oxidation, pre-lightening, and resistant hair?

Chapter 14 Makeup

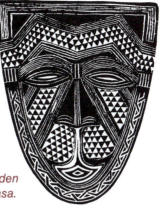

Design on Kuba carved wooden cosmetic box, Congo-Kinshasa.

After you have mastered this chapter, you will be able to:

1. List the primary, secondary, and tertiary colors.
2. Define "monochromatic colors."
3. Give the basic shades of Black skin.
4. Describe the effect makeup should have.
5. Describe the purpose of foundation.
6. Explain the shades of blush that should be considered for use on Black skin.
7. Demonstrate the procedure for eyeshadow application.
8. Explain what mascara is designed to do.
9. Give the procedure for eyeliner application.
10. Name the forms of eyebrow color used by professional makeup artists.
11. List the lipstick colors that are complementary to Black skin.

INTRODUCTION   As a makeup artist, you must be aware of the various shades of color found in the Black race and the makeup types and colors that best complement these skin tones. In this chapter you will learn how to expertly guide your client to the proper makeup selection as well as how to apply makeup in an attractive and professional manner.

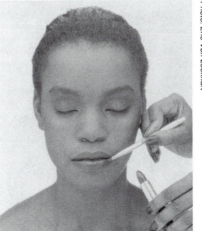

Photo: Eric Von Lockhart

COLOR THEORY	Correct selection and application of makeup tones and shad start with a basic knowledge of color theory.	

Primary Colors Red, yellow, and blue are called **primary colors**. They cann be reproduced through the mixing of any other colors. All the oth colors of the spectrum are developed from these three colors. Wh all three primary colors are mixed in equal proportions, black is result. When they are mixed together in unequal proportions, a sha of brown results.

Secondary Colors When you mix equal proportions of any two of the primary colo you get **secondary colors**. When you mix red and yellow you g **orange**. Yellow and blue mixed together yields **green**, and blue a red combined produces **violet**. So, the three secondary colors a orange, green, and violet.

Tertiary Colors When you mix equal proportions of a primary and a seconda color, you develop **tertiary color**. The tertiary colors are: **red-orang yellow-orange, yellow-green, blue-green, blue-violet**, and **re violet** (Figure 14-1).

Color Wheel

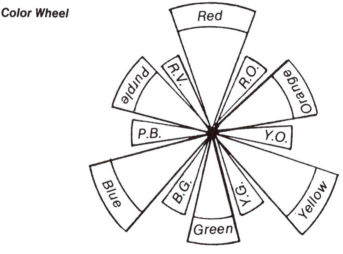

Figure 14-1.

Red	*Yellow*	*Bl*
Red + Yellow = Orange	*Yellow + Blue = Green*	*Blue + Red = Vio*
Yellow + Green *= Yellow-Green*	*Blue + Green* *= Blue-Green*	*Blue + Violet* *= Blue-Violet*
Red + Violet *= Red-Violet*	*Red + Orange* *= Red-Orange*	*Yellow + Orange* *= Yellow-Orange*

Complementary Colors　　The pairs of colors opposite each other on the color wheel are called **complementary colors.** For example, violet is the complementary color of yellow. Complementary colors are always made up of a primary and secondary color. When the colors that make up a complementary pair are placed side by side, they accent each other. When they are mixed together, however, they make a shade of brown. So, red and green side by side are holiday bright; but red and green mixed together make a neutral brown.

COLOR VOCABULARY　　Following are definitions of the various forms of color that the makeup artist must know and be able to differentiate between.

Hue　　Hue is the characteristic of colors that permits them to be classed as red, yellow, green, blue, orange, violet, and so on; color as the eye sees it.

Value　　Value is the degree of lightness or darkness of a color; for example, light brown, medium brown and dark brown. On the color wheel, lighter colors are higher in value and darker colors are lower in value.

Intensity　　Intensity is the brightness or depth of a color according to the composition of the material used. For example, an eye shadow that has been pearlized will glow, having a higher intensity than a matte shadow, which has a dull appearance.

Shade　　Shade describes the deepening of a color from its original state. For example, navy blue is a shade of blue. It is created by adding black to blue.

Tint　　Tint describes the lightening of a color. It is produced by adding white to the original hue. For example, white added to red makes pink. Pink is a tint of red.

Temperature　　**Temperature** is the warmth or coolness of a hue. Certain colors, such as red, orange, and yellow, are considered warm. Other colors, such as blue, violet, and green, are considered cool.

Monochromatic Colors　　**Monochromatic** *(mon-o-kroh-MAT-ik)* colors are the different shades and tints within one color. For example, the colors between pale pink and wine are the monochromatic colors of red.

Achromatic　　**Achromatic** *(AY-kroh-MAT-ik)* is the absence of color. Black, white, and gray are achromatic.

COLORS OF BLACK SKIN　　The expressions of color found in the Black race range from the ivory color of almonds to the density and depth of ebony wood. The skin of the Black client should be considered an asset by the makeup artist because it is complemented by more colors than the skin of clients of any other race. There is such a vast gradation in the color tones of Black skin that it could almost be described as *monochromatic*.

165

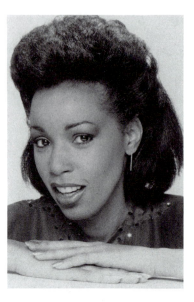

Basic Shades   There are approximately twenty-five to thirty shades of dark ski[n]. Following is a chart listing seven basic categories of Black skin col[or] in which these numerous shades fall, with the predominant undertor[e] in each color also noted.

SHADES OF DARK SKIN

Skin Color	Undertones
Cream	Yellow
Tan	Yellow
Olive	Yellow
Copper	Red
Earth brown	Yellow
Dark red brown	Red
Ebony	Deep red into blue

The color of a client's skin, eyes, and hair must all be taken in[to] consideration when deciding which makeup colors will best enhanc[e] that particular client's looks.

MAKEUP FOR BLACK SKIN   Makeup for Black skin should only enhance, not change, the loo[k] of a healthy, blemish-free skin. Each face is individual and uniqu[e]. Therefore, makeup must be personalized for each client. What ma[y] look beautiful on one face might not be attractive on another. A numb[er] of makeup artists mix their own colors to be applied to Black sk[in] in order to achieve the desired shade. However, many cosmet[ic] manufacturers offer a full range of makeup colors specifical[ly] formulated for Black skin tones. Finally, makeup should compleme[nt] the clothing worn by the client or be neutral enough not to detra[ct] from the colors of the clothes.

Note: Makeup should only be applied to thoroughly cleansed and moisturized skin.

FOUNDATION   Foundation is used to even, tone, or enhance the client's skin. You will have to use your foundation to blend uneven pigmentation for a smooth color effect. The color of the foundation should match the color of the client's skin as closely as possible. Following is a general chart that gives some basic guidelines when choosing foundation color for Black clients.

> **Note:** In cases of severe uneven pigmentation, a cover-up cream might be needed to even the skin tone before applying foundation.

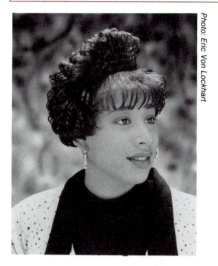

Photo: Eric Von Lockhart

SKIN AND FOUNDATION COLOR CHART

Skin Color	Foundation Color
Cream	Rosy beige
Tan	Match or coordinate with natural skin tones
Olive	Beige to even color
Copper	Medium to dark beige
Earth brown	Match or coordinate with natural skin tones
Dark reddish brown	Natural or beige to tone down red
Ebony	Match or coordinate with natural skin tones

It is important to test the foundation color before doing a full application on the client. Dab a little of the color on the jawline and blend to be sure it is compatible with the individual's coloring. Blend carefully between the jaw and the neck so that a line of demarcation does not show. Foundation that is too light for a particular skin tone will make your Black client's face appear ashy (gray).

> **Note:** It might be necessary to use two different colors on various parts of the face in order to even out your client's complexion.

Foundations come in different textures such as liquids, creams, gels, sticks, and cake forms. The liquid type of foundation is extremely popular because it gives good coverage, is easy to apply, and gives a healthy, natural look to the skin. Liquid foundation can be used successfully on almost all types of skin because the base of the liquid foundation is usually an emulsion of water and oil that spreads easily. It is sometimes referred to as a water-base foundation. Souffle makeup (lightly whipped) is light in texture and comes in jars or in mousse form. Like the liquid foundation it can be used on all types of skins. It is sometimes formulated to give extra coverage without feeling heavy on the face. An oil-based foundation is heavier in texture than souffle foundations. It feels oily to the touch and only a small amount is needed to give good coverage. The container should be shaken before use because the oil separates from the pigment. Cream and stick foundations are usually too heavy for oily skin. Cake foundation is a dry makeup that must be applied with a damp sponge; it gives good coverage but can be drying. It is better to use a water-based as opposed to oil-based makeup on Black skin that is oily.

To apply foundation: Use either the fingers or a damp silk makeup sponge. Dot foundation on the forehead, nose, cheeks, above and below the eyes, and on the ears. Stroke the foundation sparingly and evenly over the entire face and around the neckline. Use gentle upward and outward motions (Figure 14-2). Blend carefully near the hairline and remove excess foundation with a sponge or cotton. After foundation is applied, more coverage might be needed in some areas of the face, such as around the nose. In this case a small amount of foundation may be applied with the fingertips. The extra coverage will blend in with the thin, sheer film of foundation already applied.

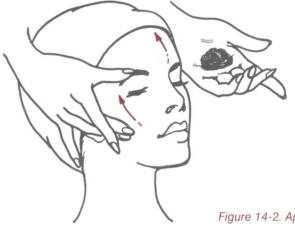

Figure 14-2. Applying foundation.

Note: To set foundation, apply translucent face powder to the client's face with either a soft powder brush or cotton puff pressed against the face. Do not use a wiping motion—you will remove traces of the foundation. Avoid using a colored face powder—it might turn orange as it absorbs oil from the face.

BLUSH OR ROUGE   Almost all Black skin tones will be complemented by the use of cheek color. When the client and cosmetologist agree that the application of blush or rouge will enhance the client's appearance, then shades of plum, wine, bronze, or umber (medium brown) should be considered. They add warmth and character to the overall look of the makeup. Avoid reds, pinks, and oranges because they are bound to look artificial on most of your clientele.

Blush comes in powder, liquid, cream, or gel form. The powder form works well on oily skin, and the cream and gel form are easy to apply. To apply liquid, cream, or gel blush: Dab a small amount of the selected blush or rouge high on the cheekbone and blend carefully with fingers or sponge in an upward and outward motion toward the temples. To apply powdered blush: Pick up a small amount of color on a soft powder brush and sweep the color from high up on the cheek bone, up and out into the hairline toward the temple.

Never apply blush on cheeks lower than the tip of the nose.

EYESHADOW   The best eye shadows for dark skin are deep and/or vibrant. Pastels will look pale and washed out on most of your Black clients. To best enhance your client's looks, choose vibrant jewel tones in blue, green, purple, and wine. Other flattering, less vivid colors are shades of gray, navy blue, muted green, and purple.

Eyeshadow comes in powder, cream, pencil, crayon, or liquid form. Powder is long lasting, a benefit to the client with oily skin. Crayons and pencils are easy to use, as is the powder. Following is one basic way to apply powdered eyeshadow (Figures 14-3—14-7).

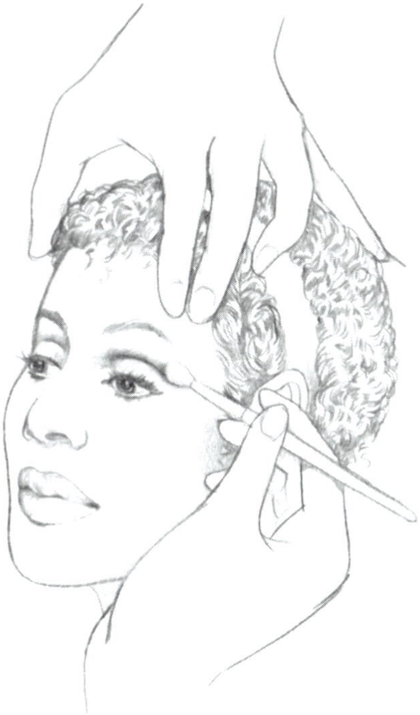

Figure 14-3. With a brush or sponge-tipped applicator, apply the color at the base of the lashes up to the crease line of the eyelid. Sometimes a deeper eye shadow color pencil is desired in place of the eyeliner.

169

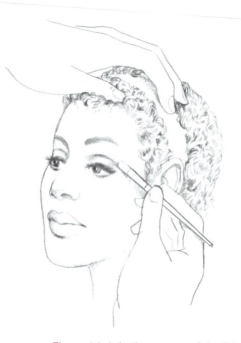 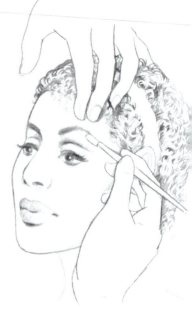

Figure 14-4. In the crease of the lid, apply a darker contouring color such as wine or dark brown. The contouring color should become lighter as it is blended closer to the eyebrows.

Figure 14-5. Directly under the brow, apply a highlighting color such as gold. The lighter color is blended into the contouring color leaving no line of demarcation. The colors should seem to flow one into the other. As fashionable colors change, the makeup artist should experiment with new styles and color combinations.

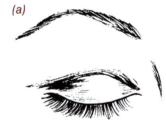 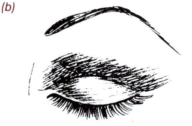

(a) (b)

Figure 14-6. Show the fold with no color showing (a) and the eye after color has been brushed higher on the lid (b).

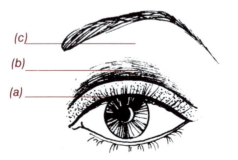

(c)_____

(b)_____

(a)_____

Figure 14-7. The basic rules to remember when applying eye shadow are shown here. (a) The main color is applied on the eyelid. (b) The contour or shading color is applied in the crease of the eyelid. (c) Highlighting is done underneath the brow.

MASCARA   Mascara is designed to make lashes appear thicker, longer and darker. Black mascara will be the most effective on your Black client. Mascara comes in cake or liquid form. The liquid form comes with an applicator wand and is more popular than the cake form, which involves the use of a small brush moistened and skimmed over the mascara cake before being stroked on the lashes. The advantage of cake form mascara is that you can more easily control the amount of mascara applied to the lashes.

Following is a basic procedure for application of mascara (Figures 14-8 and 14-9).

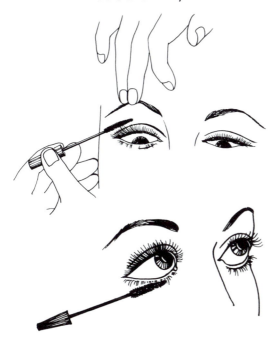

Figure 14-8. When applying mascara to the upper lashes, the client is asked to look down. The lid is lifted with the fingers for easier application. A thin coat of mascara is applied to the top and then to the underside of the lashes. It is better to build the thickness of the mascara with several light applications rather than apply a heavy coat with one application. A clean brush is used to remove excess mascara.

Figure 14-9. To apply mascara to the bottom lashes, the client is asked to look up. The bottom lashes are shorter so it will be easier to apply the mascara with just the tip of the brush. Move the brush back and forth across the lashes, then straighten them with the tip of the brush.

EYELINER   Black, charcoal gray, deep blue, deep green, and dark brown are all excellent colors to use when applying eyeliner to your Black client. Liner accentuates the eye, changes its shape, and makes the eyelashes appear thicker. Eyeliner comes in cake, soft pencils, and liquid form. Most makeup artist prefer to use the cake and an eyeliner brush.

Following is a basic procedure for applying eyeliner. Make sure the eyelids are dry and free of oil before the liner is applied. With the client looking downward, place one or two fingers on the eyelid to help hold the eye steady in case the client should blink (Figures 14-10 through 14-12).

Figure 14-10. Draw a fine line as close to the base of the lashes as possible. When the line is about two thirds across the width of the eye, start lifting the line slightly. To line the bottom lid, keep the liner only on the outer half of the lid and close to the lash growth. The cotton-tipped swabs are used to correct mistakes or to clean off excess liner. The two ends of the liner should not be brought together. The small open space at the outer end of the eye makes it look larger. When the eye is surrounded entirely by a rim of liner, the eye will appear smaller and the makeup will look too harsh and theatrical.

Correct

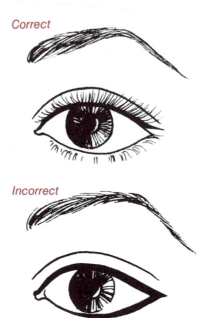

Figure 14-11. This illustration shows the correct application of eyeliner with the end slightly extended.

Incorrect

Figure 14-12. The eye is completely rimmed with liner. This causes the eye to appear smaller and the makeup too obvious.

EYEBROW COLOR   The professional makeup artist will use either an eyebrow pencil or eyebrow powder applied with a brush to create a natural look on the client. Liquid eyebrow color looks very artificial and should be avoided. Colors complementary to your clients include dark brown, charcoal gray, and sable. When color is applied to brows with a pencil, the pencil should have a fine point. Always use a pencil that has been freshly sharpened with a sanitized sharpener (Figures 14-13 through 14-19).

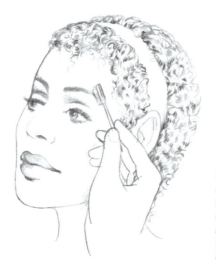

Figure 14-13. Before the application of eyebrow color, an eyebrow brush is used to remove any makeup on the brows. The brows may be brushed upward and then across in the direction of the hair growth.

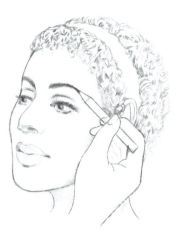

Figure 14-14. Brow color should be applied with light, hairlike strokes. When brows are sparse, a fine-pointed pencil is used to sketch in fine, hairlike strokes to resemble real brow hair. It takes practice to create the illusion of real brow hair.

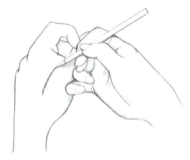

Figure 14-15. The beginning makeup artist might want to practice sketching eyebrows on the back of his or her hand until it becomes easy to create natural-looking brows.

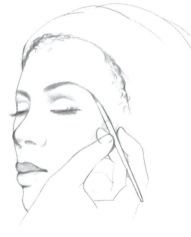

Figure 14-16. Brush-on brow color is easy to apply and works well when little corrective work needs to be done on the brows.

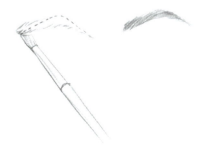

Figure 14-17. Once you have determined where the high point or apex for the brow should be, it is easy to reach this point by starting the brow color application on the underside of the brow. Stroke the color in a straight line directly up to the high point of the brow, then sweep the color outward toward the temple. Once the high point has been achieved, fill in the rest of the brow.

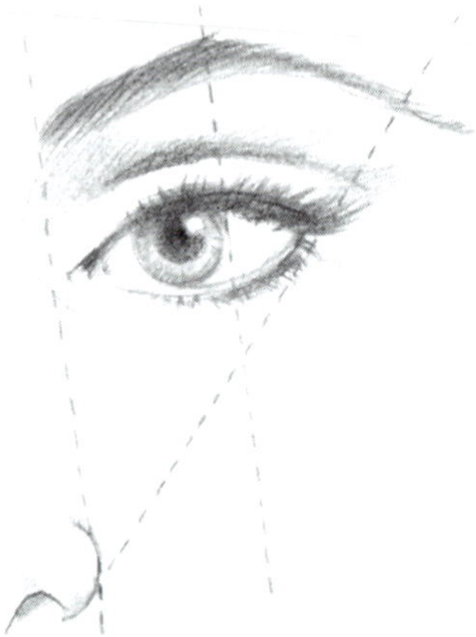

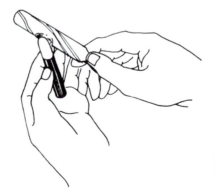

Figure 14-18. Keep in mind that for most clients, the brow will start directly above the inside corner of the eye and extend no farther outward than an imaginary line from the nostril past the outer corner of the eye. For a more dramatic or evening effect in eye makeup, the brow is sometimes extended outward. This is especially true when the eyeshadow has also been extended outward for a more dramatic effect.

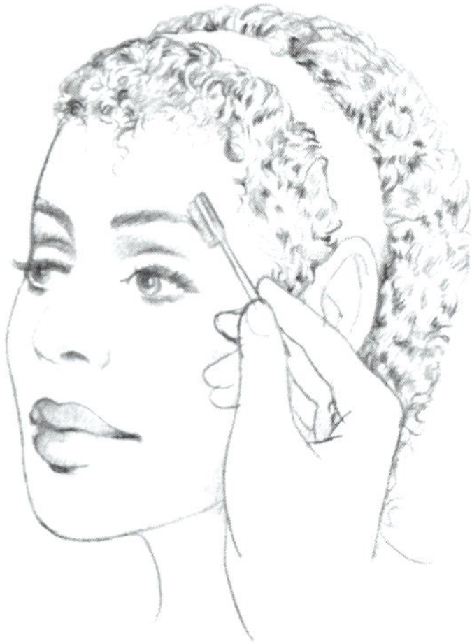

Figure 14-19. Once brow color has been applied, the brows are brushed lightly with a clean brow brush to remove excess color and give a soft, natural look to the brow.

LIP COLOR   Both lip liner and lipstick are an important part of your client's finished look. Lip liner may be applied with pencil or brush. When choosing lip liner, make sure the shade is darker than the lipstick that will be used to fill in the lips. Some lip liner shades suitable for the Black client include mahogany, dark brown, and dark red. Complementary lipstick colors to use include wine, deep red, mahogany, deep coral, red-brown, and russet. Avoid pinks and oranges when choosing lip color for the Black client, because they look unflattering against most Black skin tones. To ensure sanitation, remove lip color from the side of the stick with a spatula, then apply with a lip brush (Figures 14-20 and 14-21).

Figure 14-20. Removing lip color with a small, metal spatula.

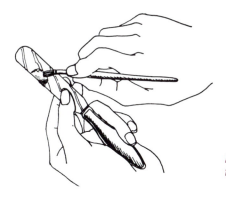

Figure 14-21. Picking up color from the spatula with a lip brush.

Procedure   Following is a basic procedure for applying lip liner and lipstick. Be guided by your instructor whose method may be different.

The client should first be asked to relax, stretch, and part her lips into a slight smile. Some makeup artists find it helpful to use the little finger on the chin to steady the hand while lining and filling in the lips. Apply lip outline to the upper lip first. Start the line at the corner of the mouth away from you. Draw the line in toward the center of the lip. Draw the line from the corner near you to the center of the lip to meet the other line. Be sure the upper curves of the lips are even. Follow the same application procedure for the lower lip (Figure 14-22). Lips may be outlined with either a lip pencil or brush. The color of the lip liner should coordinate with the lipstick being used (Figure 14-23).

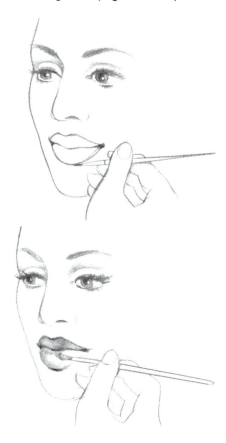

Figure 14-22. When a lip brush is used to outline the lips, the bristles are flattened so that only the edge of the bristles and the tip of the brush are used to line the lips. The flat side of the brush would make the line too thick.

Figure 14-23. After the lips have been outlined, the lipstick is filled in. The lips may be blotted, if desired, and a gloss applied to give a moist look. Attempting to alter the size and shape of your client's lips with lip color gives artificial and unattractive results. If your client is truly unhappy with the appearance of her lips, suggest to her that she use a colorless gloss that will keep her lips moist without drawing attention to them.

QUESTIONS FOR REVIEW

1. What are the primary, secondary, and tertiary colors?
2. What is the definition of "monochromatic colors"?
3. What are the seven basic shades of Black skin?
4. How should makeup affect Black skin?
5. What is foundation used for?
6. What shades of blush should be considered for Black skin?
7. How is eye shadow applied?
8. What is mascara designed to do?
9. How is eyeliner applied?
10. What forms of eyebrow color are used by the professional make artist?
11. Which lipstick colors are complementary to Black skin?

Index